Horse Genetics, 2nd Edition

D1710531

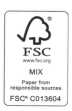

FSC
www.fsc.org
MIX
Paper from
responsible sources
FSC® C013604

Horse Genetics, 2nd Edition

Ernest Bailey
M.H. Gluck Equine Research Center
University of Kentucky
Lexington, Kentucky, USA

and

Samantha A. Brooks
Department of Animal Science
Cornell University
Ithaca, New York, USA

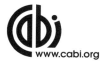

www.cabi.org

CABI is a trading name of CAB International

CABI
Nosworthy Way
Wallingford
Oxfordshire OX10 8DE
UK

Tel: +44 (0)1491 832111
Fax: +44 (0)1491 833508
E-mail: info@cabi.org
Website: www.cabi.org

CABI
38 Chauncey Street
Suite 1002
Boston, MA 02111
USA

Tel: +1 800 552 3083 (toll free)
Tel: +1 (0)617 395 4051
E-mail: cabi-nao@cabi.org

A catalogue record for this book is available from the British Library, London, UK.

Library of Congress Cataloging-in-Publication Data

Bailey, Ernest (Ernest Frank)
    Horse genetics / Ernest Bailey, University of Kentucky, M.H. Gluck Equine Research Center, Lexington, KY, USA, and Samantha A. Brooks, Cornell University, Department of Animal Science, Ithaca, NY, USA. -- 2nd edition.
        pages cm
    Previous edition by Ann T. Bowling.
    Includes bibliographical references and index.
    ISBN 978-1-84593-675-4 (pbk. : alk. paper) -- ISBN 978-1-78064-329-8 (hardback : alk. paper)
    1. Horses--Breeding. 2. Horses--Genetics. I. Brooks, Samantha A., 1979- II. Bowling, Ann T. Horse genetics. III. Title.

    SF291.B63 2013
    636.1'0821--dc23

                        2012049905

ISBN-13: 978 1 84593 675 4 (pbk)
          978 1 78064 329 8 (hbk)

Commissioning editor: Sarah Hulbert
Editorial assistant: Alexandra Lainsbury
Production editor: Lauren Povey

Typeset by SPi, Pondicherry, India.
Printed and bound by Gutenberg Press Ltd, Tarxien, Malta.

Contents

Preface to 1st Edition

Basic genetics textbooks seldom mention horses. Horse breeders tell me that they cannot relate fruit flies, corn and mice to practical horse breeding. This book aims to provide a good overview of genetic principles using horses as the primary examples. I have sifted and distilled facts and ideas to provide horse breeders with relevant illustrations. While providing a basic primer, I will not oversimplify to the point of inaccuracy. Students and science professionals can confidently use this handbook as a resource.

Do not expect to read this book from cover to cover! In my years of teaching, I have found that genetics is a subject that can only be taken in small doses. When you reach your saturation point, stop for the moment to return at another time.

Browse the contents, the pictures and tables to become familiar with the material present. You may want to read only selected chapters or sections. The index may point you to several sections discussing a subject of particular interest. If you wish to read the original research papers, the reference section provides the citations to find them in a university library. You will probably want to have a general genetics textbook at hand to refresh your memory or to provide alternative and more detailed examples of basic principles.

Knowledge about horse genes lags well behind that for human or mouse, or even for genes of other domestic animals such as [the] cow, pig, sheep, and chicken. Since the horse provides only a very limited set of examples, readers keen to know more about genetics are encouraged to consult current texts in general genetics. I especially recommend the veterinary genetics textbook by Nicholas (1987) [current edition Nicholas, F.W. (2010) *Introduction to Veterinary Genetics*. Wiley-Blackwell, Ames, Iowa] for its wealth of animal examples.

You may find the contents overwhelmingly detailed about Paint horse pattern genes. The emphasis is a reflection of the many inquiries I receive from Paint breeders. Even if white spotting genes don't pertain to your breeding program, they provide examples to help you practice thinking about horse genetics. You may be disappointed that no discussion is provided on a particular subject important to your breeding program. Information specific to horse genetics comes at a price. Government-funded agriculture programs support research on food and fiber animals, not companion animals. Knowledge about horse genetics will be forthcoming in direct proportion to how much money is invested. Without money being committed to horse research by horse breeders, our understanding about genetics of humans, mice and cattle will continue to advance rapidly, but knowledge about horse genetics will only unfold slowly.

Readers of this book will find answers to many of their questions about the genetics of horses, but I hope that other questions will replace them. Learning is a continuous process that does not end with finding answers. The path of knowledge is learning to ask questions and to build new questions from the answers.

Ann T. Bowling
1996

Preface to 2nd Edition

The preface written for the first edition of this book remains pertinent, but at the same time, many new discoveries have been made since it was written. Ann Bowling wrote the first edition just when molecular genetics was beginning to be applied to horses. At that time, parentage testing was converting from blood typing technologies to DNA technologies. The mutation had been identified for one coat color gene (*Extension*) and one disease gene (hyperkalemic periodic paralysis in Quarter Horses). Scientists were beginning to construct a genetic map for the horse with hopes of making more discoveries. Indeed, a lot has happened during the intervening 18 years. The entire DNA sequence of a Thoroughbred horse was determined. Molecular genetics has been used to identify many color genes and disease genes. Molecular markers have now replaced blood typing markers for parentage testing. DNA information is providing insights on the domestication of horses and the relationships among breeds. We are beginning to identify specific DNA sequences that influence performance and behavior. Many more horses have now had their entire DNA sequence completed. Genetics has become even more interesting and more useful.

Several years ago, the publishers asked us if we could update the existing text. Initially we declined, responding that so much had happened that it would take more than a revision to produce a useful text. However, when we took a closer look at the book, we were impressed by the organization of the topics and the quality of Ann's descriptions and explanations.

We did make some changes. We deleted the chapter on gene mapping and added chapters on evolution and genomics. The organization of the color pattern chapters was changed to reflect insights gleaned from molecular genetics. The book contains a large amount of new information and concepts reflecting research during the last decade. Nevertheless, it remains a revision inasmuch as the organization is true to Ann's original plan. Her book was a thoughtful challenge to regard genetic questions as puzzle that could be addressed with a wide range of tools.

Ann was fascinated with horse genetics and loved the opportunities she was afforded at the University of California, Davis to work on all aspects of horse genetics, especially coat color and cytogenetics. She was also an enthusiastic leader in gene mapping research for up to the time of her passing; Ann passed away on 8 December 2000 as a result of a massive stroke. The stroke was a complete surprise and Ann was at work discussing research with a colleague when it occurred. However, the greater tragedy was the loss endured by her family. Ann was a wife and mother, devoted to her family. She spoke often and proudly of Michael and Lydia. Together they operated an Arabian horse breeding farm and were proud of their bloodlines and the accomplishments of their produce.

The spirit of this book reflects Ann's love of horses and genetics. It is not necessarily the one she would have written, but Ann contributed to many of the advances described in the book and enjoyed learning of accomplishments by others. We anticipate that horse breeders and owners will find the updated text useful. The material in the book includes breeding practices that are products of centuries of experience as well new information and concepts that will make horsemanship more successful for horse and rider.

The authors are very grateful to several colleagues for critical reading of chapters, especially to Drs Teri Lear and Rebecca Bellone who provided extensive help with the chapters on Cytogenetics (Chapter 13) and Leopard Spotting (Chapter 9). Many colleagues also provided images for the book and they are identified in the legends accompanying the images.

Ernest Bailey
Samantha A. Brooks
27 November 2012

1 Evolution and Domestication of Horses

The special relationship between horses and people began over 5000 years ago. The horse encountered at the dawn of domestication was already the product of more than 50 millions of years of evolution occurring across several continents (reviewed in McFadden, 1992). Changes in climate, geography and interactions with the natural flora and fauna influenced the genes and gene combinations that were successful in each generation. By the time that people encountered the horse, it had already become large, strong, fleet, and social, traits that led to the special relationship between horses and people.

Evolution and Migration of Early Equids

Earliest ancestor of horses

The earliest recognized ancestor of the modern horse belonged to a species of the clade hyracothere (an animal or fossil of the genus *Hyracotherium*). Animals belonging to this clade were small, some say the size of a small dog, and browsed leafy vegetation across a wide landscape across North America and Europe. The hyracotheres present in North America became isolated from the rest of the world when rising waters submerged the land bridges that existed between the American and the other continents 58 million years ago. The modern horse is descended from one of the species of hyracothere present in North America 58 million years ago. Yet the hyracothere gave rise to hundreds of other horse-like species that evolved and went extinct in the intervening 58 million years. Figure 1.1 illustrates the modern view of the evolutionary processes leading to the horse.

Fossil teeth

Horse teeth have been well preserved and provide us with a perspective on the changes that may have driven horse evolution (MacFadden, 2005). From the Eocene to the early Miocene periods (58–20 million years ago) horses had short crown teeth suitable for browsing on the nutritious, leafy vegetation that was characteristic of North America during that period. However, the climate changed and grasslands became common, then predominant. Coincidental with that change, paleontologists found in the fossil record from the late Miocene era a progressive change during the late Miocene showing a decrease in the number of short crown, browsing teeth. These browsing teeth were replaced, leading to replacement in the more recent fossil record with high crowned teeth adapted to grazing.

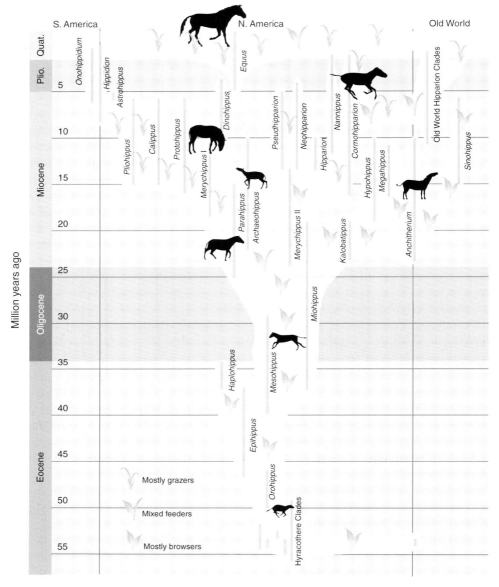

Fig. 1.1. The phylogeny, geographic distribution, diet and body sizes of the family Equidae over the past 55 million years is shown. Vertical lines represent the actual time ranges of equid genera. The first ~35 million years are characterized by browsing species of relatively small body size. The last 20 million years are characterized by genera that are primarily browsing/grazing or are mixed feeders, exhibiting wide diversity in body size. Horses became extinct in North America about 10,000 years ago but the family survived by migration across land bridges to Asia and Europe. This figure is reprinted with permission from McFadden (2005). Plio., Pliocene; Quat., Quaternary.

Aside from their impact on equid morphology, climate changes also had geographic consequences which led to the migration of many of these ancestral equid species. Between 15 and 20 million years ago, a land bridge between North America and Asia opened up and relatives of the horse (*Anchiterium, Sinohippus*) crossed into Asia. They thrived in Asia, Africa, and Europe for millions of years before becoming extinct.

Approximately 18 million years ago, extensive grasslands developed in North America and grazing became advantageous. As noted above, horses could and did evolve teeth for grazing. Furthermore, in the drier, open climates, the ancestors of horses that could travel farther and faster were favored; consequently, those with a single toe, the hoof, and other adaptations for travel became more numerous than others. Speed may have also provided protection from fleet predators. Migrations occurred a second and a third time, 5–10 million years ago, as more relatives of the horse (hipparions) crossed the land bridge to Asia and thrived for millions of years before also becoming extinct.

Meanwhile, the ancestors of modern horses continued to evolve in North America with the genus *Equus* appearing approximately 4 million years ago. Species of *Equus* crossed the land bridge to Asia, populating Asia, Africa, and Europe along with equids in the genera *Hippidion and Onohippidium*. This time, however, when the bridge closed, *Equus* became extinct in the Americas about 12,000 years ago but continued to live on the Eurasian and African continents. By this time, the other genera of Equidae had already gone extinct in Eurasia and Africa, including *Hippidion* and *Onohippidium*. It is unknown why all of representatives of *Equus* became extinct in North America but continued to live elsewhere, although species of *Equus* were among many large mammalian species that perished in the same time period. Both climate change and predation by people are suspected.

Regardless of the situation in North America, the horse continued its evolution in Asia, Africa, and Europe. Indeed, the horse did well in Europe. Cave paintings of horses in France, dated over 30,000 years ago, show that prehistoric man knew horses well. When the last Ice Age occurred, approximately 20,000 years ago, glaciers descended on northern Europe, driving all living things into southern Europe, Africa and Asia. The numbers of horses dwindled. The European horse may have been on its way to extinction as well.

Domestication of Horses

Two models exist for the domestication of animals. Model one specifies that animals were domesticated in one location and that all domestic animals of that species are descended from that original event. The second model holds that when people determined that a particular species of wild animal could be domesticated, the animals were captured and domesticated throughout the natural range of the animal. Model one predicts limited genetic variation for the species. Model two predicts wide variation. Molecular DNA studies of horses reveal wide variation and indicate that large numbers of horses were involved in domestication; whether this implies multiple independent domestication events or the continuing addition of wild horses to the population of domestic horses is not known (Vila *et al.*, 2001). Nor does the DNA sequence information tell us where or when domestication occurred. Yet archeological data does indicate a close relationship with peoples of Ukraine and Kazakhstan between 4000 and 6000 years ago. Ancient peoples routinely hunted and slaughtered horses for food (Levine, 1999). However, bit wear on teeth from the Kazakhstan sites indicated that horses may have been ridden, an activity that is unlikely without domestication (Brown and Anthony, 1998). Mare's milk residue has been also found associated with pottery, indicating that horses were kept and used for milk (Outram *et al.*, 2009). It does not appear that these people bred and raised horses. Instead, they may have captured wild horses and tamed them for domestic uses. Breeding probably came later.

A reduced number of horses would be a hardship for people who hunted horses for food. Furthermore, hunting became difficult once people developed a lifestyle based on agriculture, growing crops, and living in permanent villages. Wild animals in the vicinity of villages would have been harvested to extinction or driven off. Breeding captured horses to assure a continued supply was the next step. We do not yet know where this occurred, but this activity probably prevented the extinction of the horse and caused it to become, in evolutionary terms, one of the most successful large animals on the planet (Budiansky, 1997).

Domestication and selection

Once horses were domesticated, people had become adept at selecting horses for the characteristics they valued. This is clearly apparent in the diversity of horses that exist today. But molecular studies have provided more discrete evidence of genetic selection by prehistoric people. Ludwig *et al.* (2009) studied ancient horse DNA using genetic markers discovered for coat color variation in modern horses. They observed that DNA tests from 14,000 year old horse bones indicated that horses were uniformly bay in color. At the time of domestication, 4000–5000 years ago, genotypes for both bay and black were still apparent. In addition, DNA from those horses included DNA sequences characteristic of chestnut, tobiano and sabino. Color variation among horses therefore likely occurred coincidentally with domestication.

Summary

Fifty eight million years of evolution led to at least dozens of species of equids. The equids belonging to the genera *Hippidion*, *Dinohippus*, *Pliohippus*, *Neohipparion*, and others are all gone: extinct. Only ten equids belonging to the genus *Equus* remain. These ten remaining species are popularly known as horses (the domestic horse and Przewalski's horse), asses (the domestic donkey and Somali wild ass), zebras (Grevy's zebra, Burchell's zebra, and Hartmann's zebra), and Asiatic asses (kulans, onagers and kiangs). These are more completely described in Chapter 18. The subject of this book is the domestic horse, known scientifically as *Equus ferus caballus*.

References

Brown, D. and Anthony, D. (1998) Bit war, horseback riding and the Botai site in Kasakstan. *Journal of Archeological Studies* 25, 331–347.
Budiansky, S. (1997) *The Nature of Horses: Exploring Equine Evolution, Intelligence and Behavior*. The Free Press, New York, 290 pp.

Levine, M.A. (1999) Botai and the origins of horse domestication. *Journal of Anthropological Archaeology* 18, 29–78.

Ludwig, A., Pruvost, M., Reissmann, M., Benecke, N., Brockmann, G.A., Castanos, P., Cieslak, M., Lippold, S., Llorente, L., Malaspinas, A.-S., Slatkin, M. and Hofreiter, M. (2009) Coat color variation at the beginning of horse domestication. *Science* 324, 485.

MacFadden, B.J. (1992) *Fossil Horses: Systematics, Paleobiology and Evolution of the Family Equidea*. Cambridge University Press, Cambridge, UK, 369 pp.

MacFadden, B.J. (2005) Fossil horses – evidence for evolution. *Science* 307, 1728–1730.

Outram, A.K., Stear, N.A., Bendrey, R., Olsen, S., Kasparov, A., Zaibert, V., Thorpe, N. and Evershed, R.P. (2009) The earliest horse harnessing and milking. *Science* 323, 1332–1335.

Vila, C., Leonard, J.A., Götherström, A., Marklund, S., Sandberg, K., Lidén, K., Wayne, R.K. and Ellegren, H. (2001) Widespread origins of domestic horse lineages. *Science* 291, 474–477.

2 Basic Horse Genetics

Genes behave in very predictable ways. In fact, working with genetics can be fun and rewarding for those people who have logical thinking skills and enjoy playing sleuth. Many horse breeders will enthusiastically take on the task of learning about genetics, especially for the breed they have chosen, but interest in horse genetics is not limited to people with a breeding program. Buyers, even if not planning to breed horses, need to know what may and may not be reasonably expected. Horse owners may be fascinated to learn how one favorite steed comes to be distinctive in color, size, shape, or ability from another.

A horse show provides a good opportunity to compare characteristics that identify individual horses as belonging to a particular breed. The most conspicuous differences among breeds include color, size, gait, and carriage. Horse breeds are developed with very specific goals in mind and horses are often closely related or highly selected for the same genetic traits. Despite this powerful selection, variation continues to exist. Judges still manage to award ribbons of different colors at horse shows. Even the casual observer can discern the close relationship among, for example, Arabian horses and distinguish them from groups of Thoroughbred horses, Quarter Horses and Friesian horses. Horse breeders had an intuitive sense of genetics guiding them to create the diversity of breeds that exist today. However, the horse is not an ideal model for studying genetics.

In 1866, the Austrian monk Gregor Mendel clearly described the principles of genetics from work using with garden peas. Subsequently, scientists proved that these Mendelian genetic principles apply to the inheritance of traits in animals as well as in plants. One aim of this chapter is to describe the basic principles of Mendelian genetics using horses, not peas, as examples. But first, let us consider the nature of genes.

What Are Genes?

Until the discovery of DNA structure, the word "gene" was simply an abstract term. People used the word whenever they wanted to denote that a trait was hereditary, such as the traits of hair color, performance, or size. Genes were useful concepts, not unlike numbers or music. We cannot see concepts, but we become aware of them through experience or education. Mendel never saw a gene, yet he was able to describe the basic principles of genetics. He worked with peas just as horse breeders have worked with horses. Beginning with domestication 6000 years ago, horse breeders recognized that offspring most resembled their parents. If one wanted a gray horse, then one of the parents needed to be gray. But the inheritance of other traits, such as conformation, size, and performance, was more complex and confounded breeders. They could not discern the principles of genetics because horses were slow breeding and usually had singleton offspring. The genius of Mendel was to study plants, select a small number of traits, understand them well, then extend that concept to all of heredity.

Genes ceased being abstract concepts in 1953 (Watson and Crick, 1953). The accurate description of DNA structure as the basis for heredity created a second avenue for understanding genetics. The structure, replication, modification, and function of DNA provided a concrete basis for what had been abstract concepts. Clearly, we can best explain hereditary traits in expensive, slow-breeding species such as the horse by combining breeding studies with molecular genetics studies.

DNA

Deoxyribonucleic acid (DNA) was shown to be the chemical substance of heredity by scientists working on bacteria (Avery *et al.*, 1944). But the molecule was poorly characterized and this observation did not immediately explain how DNA worked. Since then, DNA has become iconic with genetics following the famous description of DNA structure by Watson and Crick (1953), who used chemistry and X-ray crystallography to understand DNA structure. DNA is the largest molecule found in a cell. It is also one of the simplest molecules in the cell, with only four types of basic units.

DNA structure

The nucleus of each horse cell has 64 DNA molecules. Each molecule is composed of millions of units called nucleotide bases (or just bases or just nucleotides). Only four types of bases compose DNA: adenine (referred to as A), guanine (referred to as G), thymidine (referred to as T), and cytosine (referred to as C). The bases are joined in a long, single strand which pairs with a second, complementary strand. This second strand contains a mirror image of the DNA bases found in the first. Throughout the length of this long, doubled molecule, all As in one strand pair with Ts in the other strand, and all Gs in one strand pair with Cs in the other strand. The combination is referred to as a base pair. The two strands of the DNA molecule wind around each other, with the pitch determined by the angle of the molecular bonds between each base; hence, DNA is referred to as a double helix.

DNA replication

The two-stranded structure of DNA serves two functions. Firstly, the second strand is a mirror image of the first strand, and any damage to one strand can be repaired precisely using the alternate strand as a template. We know of repair enzymes in cells that constantly monitor DNA sequences and repair any damage whenever possible. Second, the two strands provide a remarkably simple system for the replication of the DNA molecule. The two stands separate and enzymes, called DNA polymerases, create complementary strands using the original strands as templates. At the end of the process, there are two chemically identical DNA strands.

Genes coding for proteins (DNA ≥ RNA ≥ protein)

One of the major roles of DNA is to encode proteins. The process is basically the following: DNA contains a code within its sequence which is "transcribed" into another information molecule called ribonucleic acid (RNA). RNA is similar to DNA except that: (i) it is a single-stranded copy of one of the DNA strands; (ii) its structural backbone contains the sugar "ribose" rather than "deoxyribose"; and (iii) it substitutes the nucleic acid uracil (U) for thymidine wherever thymidine would have occurred based on the sequence of the DNA molecule. In transcription, one of the DNA strands is used as a template to make a complementary RNA strand such that a sequence "ATTCGAAGG" of DNA, for example, is transcribed to an RNA strand with the sequence "UAAGCUUCC". The transcribed single RNA strand is shorter than the entire DNA molecule and easily moves through the cell to join with a protein-manufacturing complex called a ribosome. Ribosomes travel down the RNA molecule, reading each set of three nucleotides and adding one of 20 amino acids according to the instructions from the genetic code.

Amino acids are small molecules which can be joined in series to create longer molecules called peptides. Two amino acids are joined to form a dipeptide, three form a tripeptide, etc. A protein can be a linear arrangement of hundreds of amino acids. There are 20 different amino acids. The differences between them reside in the side chains attached to the amino and carboxyl core of the molecule. Some of the side chains repel water, some attract water, some are basic or acid, others have the capacity to form attachments with other amino acids (disulfide bonds). All together, the combination of amino acids and their side chains cause the folding of the linear peptide and provide clefts, pockets, and receptor sites that make the protein biologically active as a structure or an enzyme. Examples of proteins include hemoglobin, immunoglobulin, and the diverse molecules making up muscle fibers, as well as the liver enzymes which detoxify blood and blood clotting enzymes which heal wounds. Mammalian genomes contain over 20,000 genes for proteins (Chapter 3).

Genetic code

DNA is an information molecule. It contains all the information necessary to transform a single cell, specifically a fertilized egg, into a complex, multicellular individual. Scientists were initially surprised that a molecule with only four basic units – A, T, G, and C – could deliver sufficient information. However, the information was found to be contained in the precise order of bases along the molecule. Each DNA molecule is millions of base pairs long with any one of the four bases possible at each position. The random permutations of base order exceed the number of animals that have ever existed! But as this is an information molecule, the order of bases is not random.

The function of a protein is based on the precise number and order of amino acids in its composition. The identity of an amino acid is determined by a set of three nucleotides. Each group of three is called a codon. As ribosomes move down the RNA molecule, they begin at a precise point which is determined by multiple factors (including the start codon, AUG), read a set of three nucleotides, then jump to the next set of three. The codons do not overlap. The triplet codes of RNA bases for amino acids are shown in Table 2.1.

Table 2.1. The genetic code based on RNA sequences read by the ribosome. The triplet codes for each of the 20 amino acids found in proteins are presented, as well as the codon signals that start and stop protein synthesis.

Amino acid/ codon signal	Codon/s	Amino acid/ codon signal	Codon/s
Alanine	GCU, GCC, GCA, GCG	Leucine	UUA, UUG, CUU, CUC, CUA, CUG
Arginine	CGU, CGC, CGA, CGG, AGA, AGG	Lysine	AAA, AAG
Asparagine	AAU, AAC	Methionine	AUG
Aspartic acid	GAU, GAC	Phenylalanine	UUU, UUC
Cysteine	UGU, UGC	Proline	CCU, CCC, CCA, CCG
Glutamine	CAA, CAG	Serine	UCU, UCC, UCA, UCG, AGU, AGC
Glutamic acid	GAA, GAG	Threonine	ACU, ACC, ACA, ACG
Glycine	GGU, GGC, GGA, GGG	Tryptophan	UGG
Histidine	CAU, CAC	Tyrosine	UAU, UAC
Isoleucine	AUU, AUC, AUA	Valine	GUU, GUC, GUA, GUG
START	AUG	STOP	UAG, UGA, UAA

Because four possible bases are used to create codons of three bases, there are 64 possible codons. As shown in Table 2.1, the 64 codons are used to signal the 20 amino acids (listed in columns 1 and 3) as well as to provide a signal to start (START) or stop (STOP) protein production. As there are 64 possibilities for 20 amino acids and two signals (start and stop), most amino acids can be encoded by more than one codon. This is referred to as "redundancy of the genetic code". For example, alanine, in the top left corner of Table 2.1, is encoded by four different codons. Only two amino acids, methionine and tryptophan, have a single codon. The amino acids with the largest number of possible codons are arginine, leucine, and serine with six each.

Technical note: sometimes DNA sequences are used to report the genetic code

A curious convention has evolved for reporting gene sequences. As described above, the genetic code is based on RNA. The information in DNA is transcribed to RNA and the information contained in the RNA sequence is translated into proteins. None the less, our molecular genetics technology is based on DNA sequences. In the laboratory, two (double)-stranded DNA is more robust than single-stranded RNA, so we usually convert RNA to DNA before sequencing. Therefore, the convention for reporting gene sequences is to use the DNA equivalent of the RNA message; in effect, this is the DNA sequence that is complementary to the one transcribed into RNA. Basically, the code is reported as shown in Table 2.1, except that all occurrences of U are reported as T.

An example is given by the bases "ATCTTCGACTTC", which form a very short part of the sequence for the gene encoding the horse skeletal muscle sodium channel alpha subunit (designated by the acronym, *SCN4A*). This base order contains information for assembling amino acids into a protein. The sequence is read in groups of three bases, starting at a precise point. For this gene in this region, the triplets are ATC, TTC, GAC, TTC. The protein sequence for these codons is reported as a string of four amino acids (isoleucine–phenylalanine–asparagine–phenylalanine). ATC always codes for isoleucine, TTC always codes for phenylalanine, GAC always codes for aspartic acid and TTC always codes for phenylalanine. This part of the protein is one very small piece that integrates into the membrane of each muscle cell.

Mutations

Sometimes DNA is altered. We know that some chemicals, UV light and radiation can alter DNA. In addition, random errors may occur when DNA strands are being copied. When this happens, the change is called a mutation. Most mutations do not cause problems. They occur in DNA regions which do not play important roles in regulating or coding for genes. Less than 3% of the DNA codes for genes. We are still determining the function of the remainder, as described in Chapter 3. However, mutations outside of protein-coding genes are less likely to have an impact on gene function.

Some mutations may make a change in the coding region which does not alter the amino acid because of the redundancy of the genetic code. With reference to Table 2.1, you can see that alanine is encoded by four different codons. The first two bases are always "GC". The third base can be U, C, A, G and still code for alanine. So changing the third base would not alter the amino acid. These kinds of mutations are called silent mutations or neutral mutations.

In other cases, sometimes the change of amino acids does not change the function of the molecule. For example, the chemical properties of glycine and alanine are similar such that a change from one to the other may not have a large effect upon protein function.

Other mutations can change the expression of the gene. For instance, a mutation in the *SCN4A* gene (described above), can cause a disease in horses. In this case, change of the second C to a G (mutation of TTC to TTG) in the short part of the sequence "ATCTTCGACTTC" results in a substitution of the amino acid leucine for phenylalanine, and is associated with hyperkalemic periodic paralysis (HYPP), an inherited muscle paralysis disease of Quarter Horses (Rudolph *et al.*, 1992).

Other kinds of mutations may entail the deletion or addition of a base. When this happens, the bases occurring in the subsequent triplet shift to a new frame according to the number of additions or deletions to the DNA. If the shift is not a multiple of three (e.g. the loss of three bases or the gain of three bases), the amino acids from that point on will be incorrectly coded by the DNA. Such mutations are called frameshift mutations. Frameshift mutations often destroy the function of a gene.

Other roles of DNA: introns and exons, and regulatory DNA sequences

All DNA sequences do not code for amino acids. The sections that code for DNA are called exons. Most proteins are encoded by (i.e. transcribed and translated from) multiple exons. The DNA sequences between the exons are called introns. Together, exons and introns comprise what we have traditionally called genes. Whenever DNA is transcribed into RNA, the entire section of introns and exons is made into RNA. Next, editing enzymes read the RNA strand and clip out introns to make the final transcript for translation into protein, called a messenger RNA (mRNA). Translation into protein at the ribosome only occurs after the introns are spliced out. The gene *SCN4A* described above, has 24 exons separated by 23 introns.

In addition to introns and exons, there are large stretches of DNA between genes, called, not surprisingly, intergenic DNA. We do not know the function of these stretches or even if they have function. But we believe these stretches of DNA may play a regulatory role in controlling gene expression. As we learn more about the importance of these regulatory pieces of DNA, we begin to ask whether these should also be called genes, even though they do not produce proteins.

Where Are Genes Found?

Genes in the nucleus

Horse genes are packaged into 64 chromosomes that are found in the nucleus of every cell. Chromosomes can be seen with the aid of a microscope and dyes that bind to DNA or to the proteins associated with DNA. The genetic information of all horses is nearly identical and, not surprisingly, horses of all breeds have the same number, size and shape of chromosomes.

When a cell starts the process of division into two daughter cells, the chromosomes condense by supercoiling from their extended state to resemble tangled spaghetti, and form into discrete rod-shaped bodies. Careful cutting and matching of stained chromosome images obtained from microscopic examination of a cell in the process of division shows that the 64 chromosomes can be arranged as a series of 32 pairs of structures. This array of paired chromosomes is known as a karyotype. The only distinguishing feature between most horse karyotypes is a difference between males and females seen in a single pair of chromosomes (the sex chromosomes), which are discussed in a later section.

Genes in mitochondria

In addition to the DNA in chromosomes, each cell has DNA in the mitochondria. Horses have 37 mitochondrial genes, all of which are dedicated to the function of mitochondria. Mitochondria are almost always inherited from the dam and these genes do not follow Mendelian principles of heredity. The special genetic behaviours of mitochondria are discussed in Chapter 16.

Behavior of Chromosomes

The conduct of chromosomes through cell life cycles is the key to the principles of Mendelian inheritance. Two types of division cycles are characteristic of chromosomes.

The first process (mitosis) occurs in all cells of the body. The second chromosome process (meiosis) is directly involved in the formation of the gametes (sperm and eggs) and occurs only in the reproductive organs or gonads (testes in males and ovaries in females).

In Fig. 2.1, the large mass near the top of the image is a large, intact nucleus. The smaller, dark staining bodies are chromosomes which have burst from another cell's nucleus. Each contains tightly coiled DNA from one of the 64 horse chromosomes. Chromosome studies are described further in Chapter 13.

Mitosis

When body cells divide, the chromosomes first replicate, then condense by tight coiling (as already described) to become the discrete chromosome elements shown in a karyotype. At cell partition, the duplicated strands separate so that each daughter cell has an exact replica of the genetic material of the original cell. This process assures that all cells of the body are genetically identical and have the normal chromosome number (the diploid number). For domestic horses, this diploid chromosome number is 64, a collection of 32 pairs of chromosomes. One chromosome of each pair has a maternal origin, the other a paternal origin.

Meiosis

Meiosis generates gametes (sperm in males and ova in females) with only 32 chromosomes (the haploid number) – only one copy from each of the chromosome pairs found in normal diploid cells. When a sperm and an ovum combine during fertilization to form a zygote, the chromosome number in the resulting cell is 64, reconstituting the diploid chromosome number and gene composition appropriate for the animal we know as the horse.

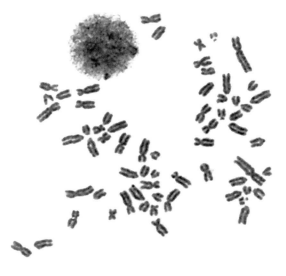

Fig. 2.1. Microscopic images of dye-stained nuclei from horse lymphocytes (white blood cells) undergoing cell division. (Image: T.L. Lear)

Chapter 2

Integral to meiosis are two programs that are directly responsible for the characteristics of gene inheritance.

- *Reduction division*, which results in the gamete receiving only one chromosome of each pair. Thus, chromosomes derived from each parent are randomly distributed through the children and on to the grandchildren. This process reassorts chromosome pairs in each generation and generates characteristic trait ratios and segregation of alleles. Mendel did not know about chromosomes, but he hypothesized this kind of process to explain inheritance.
- *Recombination*, which allows homologous maternal- and paternal-derived chromosomes to exchange sections. This crossing-over process was not part of the genetic theory hypothesized by Mendel, but is the basis for the important concept of linkage genetics.

An animal has only two copies of each gene despite the genetic input from many pedigree elements. For example, all four grandparents will provide material to the overall genetic makeup of a grandchild, although for each specific gene only two grandparents, one from the paternal side and one from the maternal side, will be represented. Certain groups of genes are likely to be co-contributed because genes are closely strung together on linear chromosomes. Meiosis ensures that genes on different chromosomes, or far apart on one chromosome, are unlikely to stay together beyond a few generations.

If this brief summary of cell division processes is not sufficient, consult a basic text on genetics for a more detailed review. For this topic, it would make very little difference for understanding the fundamental process whether a mouse, a fly or a horse was the example. From the description of the various cell and chromosome division processes, and basic to all that follows, the key point to understand is that individual genes – the units of heredity – are passed on unaltered from parent to offspring, but *the gene combinations are changed in every generation*.

The inheritance of sex

A foal's sex is determined by the genetic contribution it receives from its sire, not its dam. A clear difference between the karyotypes of males and females can be seen in one pair of chromosomes: the sex chromosomes. In the male, this pair has two different elements, while in the female the two chromosomes are indistinguishable. The sex chromosomes of the male are designated X and Y, and his configuration is referred to as XY. The sex chromosomes in the female are both X chromosome and so her pair is designated XX. The other chromosomes, apart from those involved in sex determination, are called autosomes. The members of every chromosome pair are split up during gamete formation. Every gamete receives 31 autosomes and one sex chromosome. All gametes of the female have a single X chromosome. Male gametes are an equally divided mixture of X- and Y-bearing sperm. Any ovum fertilized by an X-bearing sperm results in a filly. A Y-bearing sperm produces a colt.

Because a sperm is equally likely to contain either an X or a Y chromosome, female and male offspring are equally likely to occur. For each offspring produced, the chance of being male or female is 50%. *The sex of each offspring is independent of the sex of any previous offspring.*

Geneticists often use a simple diagram called a checkerboard or Punnett square to predict the outcome of matings (see Table 2.2). At the top right of this diagram are listed the alternative traits contributed by one parent (in this case the stallion's chromosomes, symbolized X and Y); at the top left are the alternatives from the other parent (in this case the mare, who contributes only a single X trait).

Important genetics lessons to learn from the study of sex determination are:

- Equal ratios of the trait alternatives (in this case sex) are expected among the offspring in a cross of this type. The arithmetic of genetics is that of chance. Genetics is like a game of coin tossing – with hundreds of coins in the air at once. The outcome of each coin toss is an independent event.
- The inheritance of Mendelian traits follows the inheritance pattern of chromosomes. Chromosomes occur in pairs so the genetic information for each gene is present in duplicate, but only one of the two alternatives will be transmitted, at random, from each parent to each offspring.
- Genetic contrasts between siblings could be determined solely by a difference in the contribution of one parent (for traits other than sex, this will not always be the male). When we are evaluating the inheritance of traits, our task may be made easier if we can recognize or set up situations in which trait variation is only determined by one parent (e.g. a test cross, to be discussed later), although for some types of traits this may not be possible.

The Language of Genetics

Genes and alleles

When a gene at a particular locus (the position of a gene – or a mutation – on a chromosome) has two alternative forms we call these forms alleles. Presumably, a mutation of the original gene changed the protein that it coded, resulting in a slightly different function of that protein. For example, a mutation in the gene *MC1R* resulted in a protein that causes the production of red pigment rather than black pigment. (This is the locus we called *Extension* before we knew about the mutation in *MC1R*.) This gene is discussed further in Chapter 4.

Gray is another gene which influences coat color. The *Gray* locus has two alleles, G for gray and g for non-gray. The *Gray* locus is different from the *Extension* locus, and is caused by a mutation in an entirely different gene (discussed in Chapter 7).

Table 2.2. A Punnett square showing the expected outcome of sex chromosome distribution from sire and dam to offspring, predicted to produce a 1:1 ratio of male to female offspring.

Genetic contribution from ova	Factors contributed by sperm	
	X	Y
X	XX (female)	XY (male)
Offspring proportion	50%	50%

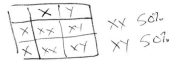

Therefore, the color gray is not allelic to the colors red or black; it is an entirely different property of hair color.

The proper assignment of traits as allelic alternatives is not always intuitively obvious. Scientists may propose allelic relationships based on information from similar traits that have been described in other animals. Novice geneticists probably will need to accept the given definition of traits as alternative alleles, but eventually they will want to understand how allelism is proven through breeding trials.

Dominant and recessive

When black parents produce a red foal, the red color factors were carried in the DNA of the black parents although they could not be seen by someone looking at the horses. The red allele is said to be recessive to black, and the black allele is the dominant alternative to red. A dominant allele is expressed even when it is carried by only one member of a chromosome pair. A recessive allele is expressed only when a dominant alternative is absent. A characteristic that is often useful to know about a recessive trait is that it will always breed true – red bred to red will always produce red. Horses that possess recessive genes which are hidden by the presence of dominant genes are called "carriers" for that gene.

A dominant allele is not necessarily associated with strength, nor is a recessive allele a sign of weakness. The terms dominant and recessive describe the relationship between alleles of one gene, not the relationship between different genes. This point *must* be understood by anyone interested in predicting genetic traits such as coat colors, as well as disease or performance genes, and will be repeatedly emphasized.

Figures 2.2 and 2.3 illustrate pedigrees in which the patterns of inheritance are characteristic of a dominant gene and a recessive gene, respectively. In these cartoon representations of a pedigree, squares represent males and circles represent females. A horizontal line joining a circle and a square represents a mating of those two individuals. The circles and squares that are attached to the vertical line joining two symbols represent offspring of that mating.

The inheritance of a dominant gene is shown in Fig. 2.2. The shapes filled in with black represent those individuals inheriting the dominant gene. There are three key points to notice: (i) all individuals exhibiting the dominant phenotype (filled-in black shape) have at least one parent with that phenotype; (ii) matings of two horses with the dominant phenotype can produce offspring without the trait; and (iii) offspring which do not inherit the trait from the parents do not exhibit the trait and cannot pass it on to their offspring. Examples of dominant genes in horses include gray coat color, tobiano coat color spotting and the disease gene for HYPP.

The inheritance pattern for a recessive gene is shown using a very similar family in Fig. 2.3. The shapes filled in with black represent those horses exhibiting the recessive trait. Again, there are three key points about recessive genes that are illustrated in this figure: (i) unaffected parents can have affected offspring; (ii) affected parents will only have affected offspring; and (iii) matings of affected horses (or carriers) to horses without the recessive gene will never produce affected offspring (illustrated here by assuming that the female mated in the third generation does not have the recessive gene and all offspring are without the recessive trait). Examples of recessive genes in horses include the red gene (*e*) for chestnut coat color and the gene for severe

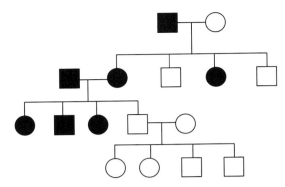

Fig. 2.2. Pedigree representation illustrating the inheritance of a dominant trait. Squares represent males and circles represent females. The black shapes represent those individuals exhibiting the dominant trait. The open or clear shapes represent those without the trait.

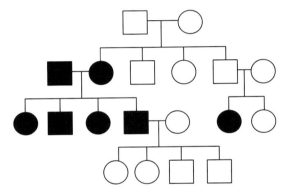

Fig. 2.3. Pedigree representation illustrating the inheritance of a recessive trait. Squares represent males and circles represent females. The black shapes represent those individuals exhibiting the recessive trait. The open or clear shapes represent those without the trait.

combined immunodeficiency disease (*SCID*) in Arabian horses. (Question: Which of the horses in the pedigree are clearly unaffected carriers? Hint: there are eight.)

Practices for Naming Genes

Names of genes and loci are always capitalized and always italicized. These practices are consistent with early conventions for genetic nomenclature; however, other conventions have diverged. At one time the practice was to always identify the locus with a single or a few letters, then represent the allele in superscript. For example the *Extension* locus was represented by the letter *E*. Dominant alleles at that locus would be represented using capital letters in superscript, e.g. the dominant allele for black pigment at the *Extension* locus was represented by E^E. The recessive alleles were represented by lowercase letters, e.g. the recessive allele for red color at the *Extension* locus was represented as E^e.

With the advances brought by molecular genetics, we have come to realize that most genes have homologues among closely related species (e.g. all mammals). A gene discovered in one species has a counterpart in another and we adopt nomenclature that reflects this comparative genetic homology. A second issue that led to an alteration in practice was the difficulties associated with using superscripts. They were difficult to reproduce on some early computers and were also more readily confused by readers because of the small print. Furthermore, the distinctions between some uppercase and lowercase letters were difficult to discern when using superscripts; an example is W^W versus W^w (*White*). Therefore, modern convention has led to dropping the superscript and representing the allele full sized, on the line, and in italics. The practice is not universal. There is no committee standard for the nomenclature of horse genes. So it behoves the reader to pay close attention to the convention used by the writer in describing those genes.

Many of the laboratories and web pages reporting the genetics of color in horses do not use superscripts. Instead, they identify the locus by name, then represent the alleles using full-sized italic letters. For example, the *Extension* locus (*E*) has two alleles, one producing black pigment and identified as *E*, and the other producing red pigment and represented as *e*. As before, the dominant alleles are represented by capital letters and recessive alleles are represented by lowercase letters.

With the advent of molecular genetics, it has been possible to identify the DNA sequence and actual gene responsible for the trait of black or red color. In Chapter 4, the *Extension* locus is described as being the gene *Melanocortin-1 Receptor* (*MC1R*). The precise DNA changes responsible for the two alleles are known and we could represent the alleles in a format reflecting the DNA strand or the changes in amino acids for the protein. However, it has been simpler and easier to continue using the conventional nomenclature of the *Extension* locus when referring to this gene in the context of coat color genetics. This is true with most of the other genes which had been identified and named before the discovery of the underlying molecular genetics.

Some writers may change the nomenclature used in an effort to increase clarity for the reader. While this may work in the short term, it will cause problems when readers compare different papers from different writers. For instance, the gene for non-dilution at the *Cream* dilution locus has been represented by different authors as *C*, *C+* and *N*. (For the record, we are referring to that allele as cr) At this point, there is no internationally recognized naming convention for horse coat color genes. Therefore, as already noted, the reader needs to pay particular attention to which locus the authors are describing and to the subsequent description of the alleles to determine the points of correspondence between papers.

A full discussion of the issues of genetic nomenclature, as well as a proposal for nomenclature guidelines for the horse, can be found in Dolling (2000).

Mendelian Ratios

Phenotype and genotype; homozygous and heterozygous

The difference between black and red coat color is due to the alleles of *Extension*, the black pigment gene, symbolized as *E*. The dominant allele is assigned a capital letter, *E*. The recessive allele is *e*. In describing the genetic traits of any animal, the genotype designates the alleles present and the phenotype specifies the external appearance resulting from the interaction of allelic pairs (see Table 2.3).

Table 2.3. Chart showing the relationship of genotype to phenotype for the different combinations of the alleles *E* and *e* of the *Extension* gene for coat color.

Genotype	Phenotype
EE	Black hair
Ee	Black hair
ee	Red hair

Nomenclature for ambiguous genotypes

The genotype of a red horse will always be *ee*. Because the black allele is dominant to the red allele, the genotype for a black horse is not readily apparent from the phenotype. Genotypes *EE* and *Ee* will both have a black phenotype (although horses may actually be bay, black or buckskin depending on the alleles present at other loci). We know that one allele is *E* because black is present. Unless we have further genetic information we cannot know whether the second allele is *E* or *e*. By convention, we list the unknown allele as a "–". A black horse of unknown parentage would be identified by the genotype as "*E–*". When both alleles in a pair are the same (*EE* or *ee*), the horse is said to be homozygous; when the pair has unlike alleles (*Ee*), the horse is said to be heterozygous.

A Punnett square shows how two black horses can produce red (chestnut) offspring and the expected proportions of black and chestnut offspring (Table 2.4).

We now have molecular tests to determine the precise genotype of a horse (see Chapter 4). But before these tests were developed, one needed to perform test crosses to determine the genotype. One way to determine which black horses are *EE* and which are *Ee* is through a test cross to an *ee* (chestnut) horse, as no direct assay for the *e* allele is available. A test cross is a mating between a homozygous recessive animal and an animal with the phenotype of the dominant allele. Such a cross provides evidence to define the genotype of an animal with the dominant phenotype. In a test cross, a homozygote *(EE)* for the dominant phenotype will never have foals of the recessive (*ee*) phenotype, but a heterozygote (*Ee*) will have foals of both the dominant and recessive phenotypes in a 1:1 ratio.

Sometimes, a pedigree or family study can help to determine genotypes that may not be obvious from the phenotype. For example, a black horse with a chestnut sire, and any black horse that produces a chestnut foal, will necessarily be *Ee*.

Ratios for lethal traits

The dominant *White* coat color gene (*W*) is one of the earliest lethal genes described for horses. Molecular genetic studies have determined several mutations that are responsible for dominant white in horses, and these are discussed in Chapter 6. A breeding study by Pulos and Hutt (1969) suggested that at least one of the mutations that causes a white coat could cause embryonic losses. In matings between white horses, both solid color (non-white) and white foals were always produced, demonstrating that the gene for white coat color (W) was dominant to the non-white gene (w). However, the ratio of white to colored foals (28:15) from matings of heterozygous white horses (Ww) did not correspond to the expected ratio of 3:1 that would be expected in matings of known heterozygotes (see Table 2.5). In this case, the results more closely approximated a 2:1 ratio. This could be explained if homozygous white (WW) offspring are lost as embryos, and only the heterozygous white and the non-white offspring make it to term, as shown in Table 2.5. Consistent with this observation, the authors of the study did not observe true-breeding white horses (homozygotes) in their herd (Pulos and Hutt, 1969).

Incomplete dominance and codominance

Occasionally, homozygous and heterozygous genotypes for a dominant trait have recognizably different phenotypes. While this is not the case for the *Extension*

Table 2.4. This Punnett square shows the results of crossing black horses heterozygous for the *Extension* gene. The cross produces black and red foals in a 3:1 ratio. The black-producing allele *E* is dominant to the red-producing allele *e*.

Genetic contribution from *Ee* mare	Offspring characteristic	Genetic contribution from *Ee* stallions	
		E	*e*
E	Offspring genotype	*EE*	*Ee*
	Offspring phenotype	Black	Black
	Proportion of offspring	25%	25%
e	Offspring genotype	*Ee*	*ee*
	Offspring phenotype	Black	Chestnut
	Proportion of offspring	25%	25%

Table 2.5. If all classes of offspring are equally viable, the proportion of white to colored offspring from matings between white horses heterozygous for the dominant *White* gene *W* is expected to be 3 white: 1 colored. If one homozygous class is lethal, then the proportion of white to colored would be 2:1. Relatively large numbers of offspring might be needed to distinguish between a 3:1 and a 2:1 ratio.

Genetic contribution from *Ww* mare	Offspring characteristic	Genetic contribution from *Ww* stallions	
		W	*w*
W	Offspring genotype	*WW*	*Ww*
	Offspring phenotype	Embryonic loss	White
	Proportion of offspring	25%	25%
w	Offspring genotype	*Ww*	*ww*
	Offspring phenotype	White	Not white
	Proportion of offspring	25%	25%

genotypes *EE* and *Ee*, which both have a black coat color, another coat color provides an example of this effect. A coat color dilution gene of horses can be used to demonstrate dosage effect – or incomplete dominance. Palominos and buckskins are heterozygous for the *Cream* allele (*CR*) of the basic color gene; they have the genotype *CRcr*. The gene action of *CR* dilutes red pigment to yellow. Hence, chestnuts with *CR* become palominos and bays with *CR* become buckskins. Cremellos are homozygous for the cream allele (*CRCR*). For cremellos, all pigment (both black and red) is diluted to a very pale cream.

In Chapters 11 and 17, we will see examples of genetic markers that are inherited as *codominant* traits. For such traits, allelic variants do not demonstrate dominant and recessive relationships, but are always co-expressed. There are no good examples among coat color or disease genes of horses, but we can identify these when we test for genetic markers. In such cases, the phenotype exactly indicates the genotype. For example, the gene for albumin has two common alleles which are detectable using a biochemical test. A genetic marker test shows that horses have two copies of the allele for A albumin or two copies of the allele for B albumin or one copy of each. This corresponds exactly to being homozygous for A or B albumins or heterozygous A and B albumins. Codominant inheritance of alleles can be used as an efficient and powerful tool for parentage testing.

Expected ratios, statistical tests and alternative models

Learning to predict and recognize simple 1:1, 1:2:1, 3:1. and 2:1 trait ratios among offspring is extremely useful for building genetic models of trait transmission. These ratios may be complicated, as we have seen, by the interactions of more than one gene, and may not be obvious unless large numbers of offspring are available. Statistical testing (e.g. the chi-square test) may be needed to determine whether the observed ratios match the expected ratios. (Consult a basic genetics or statistics text for information on how to apply such tests.)

If the data obtained do not match expected ratios, then alternative proposals need to be considered, such as:

- The trait is genetic but the hypothesized transmission mechanism is incorrect (e.g. more than one gene may be involved).
- The trait is produced by environmental influences, not genes.
- The gene shows "reduced penetrance" (i.e. the phenotype is modified by environment or other gene combinations, so that the effect of the mutant gene is not easily recognized).
- One genotypic class is lethal, so the expected ratios need to be adjusted accordingly.
- Several of these mechanisms simultaneously influence the trait expression.

It is obviously much easier and faster for an individual dog breeder to obtain statistically significant data working with litters of puppies than for a horse breeder working with a single birth per mare each year! Indeed, with rare exceptions, such as the study of dominant white by Pulos and Hutt (1969), horse breeders are unlikely to use such information. However, understanding the principles are important to understanding genetics.

Two genes and more

As the genetic makeup of every horse consists of thousands of genes, a horse breeder will want an understanding of the complex results expected from the interaction of the products of more than one gene. The now familiar Punnett square provides a model for predicting the outcome when two independently inherited traits are simultaneously considered, such as sex and black/red color (Table 2.6).

The four different genetic types of sperm can combine with the two types of ova to generate eight genotypic classes of offspring (four phenotypes). Due to chance, any particular mating of this type may never produce any red females or males, while others may have two or three of each. When data from many matings are combined and evaluated by statistical tests, the hypothesized outcomes of the random events shown in the Punnett square will be validated.

Dihybrid cross

Moving along to a slightly more complicated situation, consider a mating between dun tobianos, each heterozygous for the genes controlling the dun and tobiano patterns. Geneticists label a cross between double heterozygotes a dihybrid cross. The dun color is a dominantly inherited trait that modifies the expression of the *Extension* gene to produce horses of diluted coat color and a distinctive pattern of striping on the legs and along the back. Tobiano is a white spotting pattern inherited as a dominant trait. The phenotypic ratios among the offspring of such a cross between heterozygotes for the two genes will be 9:3:3:1 (Table 2.7). This chart does not show the interaction of these two genes with a third important color gene – *Extension*. Try your understanding of gene interaction by drawing that Punnett square with 64 possible genotypes. To help you know when you have the right scheme, the predicted number of classes is eight, with phenotypic ratios of 27:9:9:9:3:3:3:1. (Hint: the most frequent class has at least one copy of the dominant allele for each gene and the least frequent class is homozygous for the recessive alleles for each gene.) Even more

Table 2.6. Punnett square diagram showing independent assortment of two traits, gender and basic coat color of offspring for mares and stallions, both heterozygous for the black (*Extension*) color gene (*Ee*). X and Y are the sex chromosomes. *E* and *e* are allelic genes producing the black/red coat color. Each trait shows a 3:1 ratio (black to red or female to male). Considered together, the phenotypic ratios are 3:3:1:1 – 3 black males, 3 black females, 1 red male, and 1 red female.

Genetic contribution from *Ee* mares (XX)	Genetic contribution from *Ee* stallions (XY)			
	X E	X e	Y E	Y e
X E	XX *EE* Black Female	XX *Ee* Black Female	XY *EE* Black Male	XY *Ee* Black Male
X e	XX *Ee* Black Female	XX *ee* Red Female	XY *Ee* Black Male	XY *ee* Red Male

Table 2.7. Complex interaction between two genes is demonstrated in a dihybrid cross between two heterozygous dun (*Dd*) tobiano (*Toto*) horses. The dun to not-dun ratio is 3:1; tobiano to solid is 3:1. Four phenotypes in a 9:3:3:1 ratio are found among offspring – 9 dun and tobiano, 3 tobiano, 3 dun solid, and 1 solid.

Genetic contribution from mares (eggs)	Genetic contribution from stallions (sperm)			
	D TO	*D to*	*d TO*	*d to*
D TO	*DD TOTO*	*DD TOto*	*Dd TOTO*	*Dd TOto*
Color of cross	Dun tobiano	Dun tobiano	Dun tobiano	Dun tobiano
D to	*DD Toto*	*DD toto*	*Dd Toto*	*Dd toto*
Color of cross	Dun tobiano	Dun solid	Dun tobiano	Dun solid
d TO	*Dd TOTO*	*Dd TOto*	*dd TOTO*	*dd TOto*
Color of cross	Dun tobiano	Dun tobiano	Tobiano	Tobiano
d to	*Dd TOto*	*Dd toto*	*dd Toto*	*dd toto*
Color of cross	Dun tobiano	Dun solid	Tobiano	Solid

complicated examples could be constructed, but the point to be taken is that a basic understanding of the allelic actions of genes allows model building to predict the outcomes of complex interactions.

Note that in Table 2.7, the possible offspring genotypes for the two traits of dun and tobiano show the two sets of alleles that are present (e.g. *DD TOTO*) separated by a space. Sometimes though, and especially if the names of the alleles are long or complex (or because of other particular conventions), the alleles are separated by forward slashes (see Tables 8.3 and 8.4; *HYPP* alleles in Chapter 12).

Epistasis and hypostasis

Occasionally, the action of the alleles of one gene may cover up the actions of another. The masking of allelic effects that results from interaction with alleles of a gene at a different site or location on a chromosome is called epistasis, not dominance. (Dominant and recessive refer to interactions between alternative alleles from the same site.) The gene that is masked by epistasis is said to be hypostatic. The *Gray* gene is a common example of a gene with epistatic action. This is a dominant gene, meaning that only one copy is necessary for exhibition of the trait, which halts the production of pigment in hair cells within several years of the birth of horses. At birth, horses may exhibit a variety of color patterns, including chestnut, bay, tobiano, appaloosa, sabino, etc. However, when they have the *Gray* gene, they begin to lose that color and by the age of 10 usually have only white hair. The *Gray* gene (*G*) is dominant to its allele (*g*), so, as mentioned above, only one copy is necessary to produce the gray color. The mutation responsible for the gray color has been discovered and is discussed in more detail in Chapter 7. While gray horses can be impressive and are popular for parades, the gene for gray is very frustrating for breeders interested in appaloosa, pinto and many of the other coat color patterns of horses.

Linkage

Although the independent inheritance of genetic traits has been emphasized up to now, some genes will tend to be inherited together. The august monk Mendel did not envision the relationship that we now know to exist between genes and chromosomes. But to understand genetics more completely, it is necessary to expand his otherwise elegant theories to include gene linkage.

Any given gene has a particular chromosomal assignment and a place on that chromosome that we call a locus (plural: loci). Occasionally, traits of interest are on the same chromosome and tend to be inherited together more often than they are split apart: these are linked genes. Linked genes can be separated from each other as part of the normal process of chromosome recombination that occurs uniquely during meiosis. At present, the entire genome of the horse has been sequenced and we know the location and sequence of many genes of interest for the horse (see Chapter 3, Horse Genomics). Yet our understanding of the relationships of the bits of DNA to behavior, performance, and many other phenotypic characters that we value in the horse remains to be developed.

Sex-linked genes

A special case of linkage relates to genes on the X chromosome. X-linked genes are often called sex linked, to contrast them with autosomal genes, which are located on any of the other 31 pairs of horse chromosomes. Remember that males have only one X chromosome; in this case, we refer to males as being hemizygous, because they only ever have one copy of a gene from the X chromosome. Females, in contrast, may be either homozygous or heterozygous for X chromosome genes. The relationship of the X chromosome to gender has a particular impact on the ratio and occurrence of traits associated with the X chromosome. One of the genes residing on the X chromosome is important for the production of a blood clotting protein called Factor VIII. Individuals without an effective Factor VIII protein have hemophilia, a condition in which the blood will not clot and the individual can easily bleed to death. The mutation that causes the production of defective Factor VIII is recessive. A horse needs to have only one good copy of the gene for Factor VIII in order to avoid hemophilia. However, as only females have two copies of the X chromosome, they are the only ones that can be protected by the presence of a second copy of the gene. Males that inherit the mutated gene, albeit in the recessive form, will develop hemophilia. The inheritance of X-linked recessive disease-causing genes has an expression pattern that reflects the transmission of the sex chromosomes. Although it is possible for females to inherit two copies of such recessive sex-linked genes, they will have a much lower prevalence of the corresponding phenotype than the males that inherit only one copy. Of course, if the X-linked gene is lethal in males, then it will never be seen in females because a male is not going to transmit the gene to its female offspring.

Polygenic (Multiple Gene) Traits

We have come to understand genetics by the investigation of genes that have a simple effect on phenotype. Such genes affect coat color, cause diseases or are useful for parentage testing. But most traits are influenced by more than one gene. The phenotypes related to horse speed, endurance, conformation, height, behavior, and gait cannot be as easily broken down into simple dominant and recessive gene combinations. These are quantitative traits in that horses do not exhibit a simple presence and absence of the trait, but rather, exhibit a continuous range for these traits. It may be that there are many genes related to speed and the horse with the most of them is the fastest. It may be that there are different combinations of many genes that make a horse fast. We do not know. But, in practice, breeders have been studying these traits for hundreds, if not thousands, of years. In recent years, we have begun to refer to the hypothetical genes for these traits as quantitative trait loci (QTLs). Considerable work has been done to investigate QTLs for meat, milk, fiber, and eggs in other areas of the agricultural industry. With the availability of the horse genome sequence and the application of the methods developed in other species, we will begin to discover and understand QTLs in horses.

Determination of Inheritance Patterns

Genetics is responsible for much of the variation we see among horses. Applying the principles of genetics to make progress in breeding programs, or to just understand the genetics of one's own horse, can be fun. But all variation is not genetic. Before assuming that a trait has a genetic basis, other factors must be ruled out, including management, exposure to toxins, infectious diseases, and even random chance. At the beginning of every genetic study, the following questions must be addressed:

1. Are differences seen between different horse populations (breeds)?
2. Is the effect localized to one farm or region, especially without regard to breed?
3. Is there a familial aspect within a breed?

If the answer to these questions is "no", then the trait is unlikely to be hereditary.
    Consider the following:

1. Horses within a breed share the same set of genes. If a trait is caused by genes, then it is more likely to be seen in some breeds than others. Differences between breeds are a hallmark of hereditary traits.
2. If management is responsible, then there will be a farm effect. The use of contaminated feed or the appearance of toxins in the water can adversely affect reproduction and development, and sometimes may mimic a genetic basis. Management problems are difficult to determine because breeders may have unique breeding programs on individual farms. However, if the trait is hereditary, it may have been seen on other farms with horses of similar pedigrees.
3. If the trait is hereditary, then there may be lines within a breed that are affected as well as lines that are not. Breeders may already have a sense of the stallions that are carriers for good and bad traits. This can be a serious issue, because casting aspersions on breeding stock can be deleterious to the commercial interests of breeders. Hence, it becomes very important to determine the precise cause of a trait and to devise ways to manage it without losing access to valuable breeding stock.

Components of genetic research include:

- Searching the scientific literature to find a well-described candidate gene that causes similar clinical and pathological characteristics in other mammalian species.
- Collecting pedigrees of horses that express the trait so as to search for relationships.
- Collecting tissue samples (blood or hair roots) to store for possible future genetic marker research (especially to look for DNA markers).
- Collecting offspring data from breeders to suggest the pattern of trait transmission.
- Designing matings and performing crosses to test genetic hypotheses, which is an essential, major money-consuming aspect of any research proposal.

The main patterns of inheritance (trait transmission), can be summarized as follows.

- An *autosomal dominant* trait will show direct transmission from parent to off-spring (except in the unlikely event the trait has just appeared as a new mutation). About 50% of offspring of both sexes will have the trait. If the trait is a disease problem, normal offspring of affected parents when mated to a normal mare or stallion will produce only normal foals. The trait will generally be rare and confined to a single breed. It will be frequent in the family in which it occurs, even if the family shows little inbreeding.
- An *autosomal recessive* trait will initially probably be seen in both sexes as a result of matings between horses without the trait (usually related). It will generally be confined to one breed or to closely related breeds. This kind of genetic trait can appear to skip generations. When animals with the trait are mated together, all the offspring will show the trait. The trait will be more frequently seen in inbred families.
- An *X-linked recessive* trait is generally obvious from an apparent association with males, but is not a trait that is necessarily associated with sexual characteristics.
- A *polygenic* trait will: (i) be most frequent among related horses; (ii) shows exceptions to the dominant/recessive modes of inheritance; and (iii) is not usually confined to a single breed. Polygenic traits often show a continuous range of variation, ranging from normal to slightly affected to extremely affected. Examples of such traits in humans include diabetes and heart disease; for horses, conformation traits and performance traits behave as polygenic traits.

Summary

We have a much richer vocabulary to discuss genetics than was available to Gregor Mendel. But genes remain abstract concepts discussed using words such as dominant, recessive, reading frame, double helix and Punnett square. Nevertheless, these concepts are useful to make us more successful horse breeders.

References

Avery, O.MacLeod, C. and McCarty, M. (1944) Studies on the chemical nature of the substance inducing transformation of pneumococcal types: induction of transformation by a desoxyribonucleic acid fraction isolated from pneumococcus type III. *Journal of Experimental Medicine* 79, 137–158.

Dolling, C.H.S. (2000) Standardized genetic nomenclature for the horse. In: Bowling, A.T. and Ruvinsky, A. (eds) *The Genetics of the Horse*. CAB International, Wallingford, UK, pp. 499–506.

Pulos, W.L. and Hutt, F.B. (1969) Lethal dominant white in horses *Journal of Heredity* 60, 59–63.

Rudolph, J., Spier, S., Byrns, G., Rojas, C., Bernoco, D. and Hoffman, E. (1992) Periodic paralysis in Quarter Horses, a sodium channel mutation disseminated by selective breeding. *Nature Genetics* 2, 144–147.

Watson, J.D. and Crick, F.H. (1953) Molecular structure of nucleic acids; a structure for deoxyribose nucleic acid. *Nature* 171, 737–738.

3 Horse Genomics

Genes do not function alone. Most genes exist, function, and have effects within a network of thousands of other genes. While we consider genetics as the study of single genes, genomics is the study of all genes in an individual or population. Until recently, we only studied genes one at a time. We did not have the ability to study or use genomics to aid our genetic studies. In fact, we did not even know how many genes there were. That changed with the advent of the human genome project.

Genome Projects

The Human Genome Project began in 1990 with the goal of sequencing all of the DNA that exists in a human cell by 2005. It was a bold plan. At that time, we could sequence stretches of DNA containing thousands of bases, but the entire genome contained 3 billion base pairs (bp); today it would be like planning manned flight to Mars within the next 15 years. The technical challenges were awesome. The capacity to organize and sequence 3 billion bp of DNA did not exist; the amount of information generated would exceed the capacity of computers and computer programs to analyze and organize. Clearly, the initial task for the human genome project was to invent new technologies. By 1997, only 3% of the human genome had been sequenced. However, DNA sequencing machines were invented through the process that led to completion of the first draft by 2001, and of the entire project by 2003, some 2 years ahead of schedule (International Human Genome Sequencing Consortium, 2001; Venter *et al.*, 2001).

The new technologies invented in connection with the Human Genome Project made the investigation of genomic DNA inexpensive and relatively easy to perform. Indeed, some students in high school biology classes now perform laboratory exercises in which they sequence short stretches of DNA. Its reduced costs placed molecular genetics technology within reach of scientists working on livestock, including horses. Discoveries resulting from the Human Genome Project had already made it clear that the future of applications of agricultural research entailed having a detailed gene map or even a whole genome sequence for agriculturally important animals.

In October 1995, a horse genome mapping workshop was held in Lexington, Kentucky to make a plan for mapping the horse genome – the Horse Genome Project (see Websites section for URL). At the time, no single laboratory had the resources to map the horse genome. Therefore, a group of approximately 100 scientists from 25 laboratories around the world met at annual workshops, shared information, and methodically created a gene map that led to many discoveries that are part of this volume. More significantly, the existence of the research community and the quality of the developing horse gene map led the National Human Genome Research Institute to sequence the horse genome in 2006.

Differences between a genome map and a genome sequence

Initially, DNA sequencing the horse genome did not seem possible. It was expensive. Consequently, the scientists working on the horse simply identified the commonalities between the human genome and the horse, then used information from the Human Genome Project to predict the organization and sequence of genes in the horse. Toward that goal, several techniques were used to create various types of maps:

- synteny maps (Bailey *et al.*, 1995; Caetano *et al.*, 1999; Shiue *et al.*, 1999) – maps localizing genes to specific chromosomes
- linkage maps (Penedo *et al.*, 2005; Swinburne *et al.*, 2006) – maps based on family studies showing gene order and distance between them
- cytogenetic maps (Bowling *et al.*, 1997; Lear *et al.*, 2001, Milenkovic *et al.*, 2002) – maps based on microscope images localizing genes to chromosomes
- zoo-FISH chromosome painting maps (Raudsepp *et al.*, 1996) – maps comparing gene organization between different species (see Chapter 13)
- radiation hybrid (RH) maps (Raudsepp *et al.*, 2010) – maps similar to synteny maps but having a resolution that shows gene order and distance between genes.

The net effect was of the utilization of these techniques was overlapping sources of evidence that identified chromosome locations, gene orders, and distance between genes. Taken altogether, this information was collated and assembled to identify landmarks on horse chromosomes for comparison with the organization of genes that had been identified for humans. Figure 3.1 illustrates a genome map for horse chromosome 3 (ECA3) and compares its organization with that of two human chromosomes (HAS4 and HSA16).

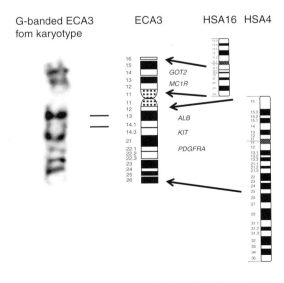

Fig. 3.1. Image of a G (Giemsa)-banded horse chromosome 3 (ECA3), an ideogram of ECA3, and positions of genes or DNA markers, and comparison with the organization of genes on human chromosome 4 (HSA4) and 16 (HSA16).

Chapter 3

This figure illustrates several important points. Firstly, the organization of genes is not identical for horses and humans. This should at once seem obvious because people have 46 chromosomes while horses have 64 chromosomes, so a one-to-one correspondence cannot exist. Second, human genes and horse genes appear to be homologous. Many horse DNA sequences showed 80–98% identity to DNA sequences for genes already identified in humans. Third, the organization of genes was similar. From Fig. 3.1, it is apparent that ECA3 does not have a precise equivalent in humans, though the long arm of ECA3 appears to have the same genes as the top half of human chromosome 4 (HSA4) and the short arm of ECA3 appears to have the same genes as the bottom arm of human chromosome 16 (HSA16). An assumption of complete homology leads us to predict the remaining genes on ECA3. The human genome is an excellent model for the horse genome. The horse genome map guides us in our use of the human genome sequence to predict horse sequences.

Completion of the Human Genome Project and realization of horse genome sequencing

Once the human genome sequence was completed, the information from it generated more questions. One major surprise was the number of genes. In 1990, scientists speculated that the human genome might contain 100,000 to 300,000 genes coding for proteins. When the sequencing was completed and the DNA analyzed, the number of genes was only around 20,000. In fact, all mammals appear to have between 19,000 and 24,000 genes. How could the diversity and function of complex animals be directed by a mere 20,000 genes, most of which were shared between species?

Another observation was that only 2% of the human genomic DNA was for genes. The remaining 98% of the DNA did not have a known function. Taken together, these two observations led to the hypothesis that the genetic diversity that comprises the differences among and within species is a result of the regulation of genes by the 98% of the non-protein coding DNA. How could this hypothesis be tested?

Sequencing another human would produce the same pattern but not shed light on the function of the non-protein coding DNA. But comparing sequences among mammals might identify non-protein coding DNA that was conserved among all mammals. Once those regions were identified, experiments could be conducted to determine their function in the genome. Therefore, the National Human Genome Research Institute (NHGRI, see Websites section for URL) began sequencing a wide range of animals representing the diverse branches of phylogeny and evolution. Although the purpose was to benefit human health research, the plan was a major boon for the equine.

Horse Genome Sequencing

The sequencing of Twilight's genome

The horse genome was sequenced at the Broad Institute of MIT and Harvard at Boston, Massachusetts (see Websites section for URL) as part of a project by the

NHGRI. A Thoroughbred mare, named Twilight, was chosen for genome sequencing. Twilight was part of a research horse herd at Cornell University in New York state. DNA was isolated from her white blood cells in 2005 and sent to the Broad Institute in Boston for sequencing. Pieces of her genome were sequenced and made publically available for research in 2006, subsequently followed by the publication announcing the annotated genome (Wade *et al.*, 2009). Information, including the completely assembled DNA sequence, annotations for genes and comparisons with the genomes of other species can be found on the websites of the following three institutions (see Websites section for URLs): the Genome Center at University of California at Santa Cruz; ENSEMBL – a joint project between EMBL–EBI (the European Bioinformatics Institute of the European Molecular Biology Laboratory) and the Wellcome Trust Sanger Institute in Cambridge, UK; and the National Center for Biological Information (NCBI) in Washington, DC.

The genome assembly for Twilight contained 2.43 billion DNA bp. The next step was to annotate the sequence, specifically utilizing existing information to identify the genes of the horse. However, little information was available about the genes expressed in the horse. Therefore, the horse genome was annotated using genomic information from other species, especially the human. The DNA sequences were analyzed by ENSEMBL and NCBI, with estimates of 20,322 genes by ENSEMBL and 17,610 genes by NCBI (Coleman *et al.*, 2010). The different numbers from the two annotations, were the result of the different methods that each group used to validate genes, but it is generally believed that there are over 20,000 genes. Furthermore, these estimates will change as we learn more about horse genes. Indeed, we still do not know precisely the number of human genes despite vastly more research in this area.

The DNA sequence is now available for all 31 autosomes and the X chromosome for horses, though the DNA sequence for the entire Y chromosome remains incomplete at the time of writing. As noted in Chapter 2, female mammals have two X chromosomes, while males have one Y and one X chromosome. Twilight was a female, so her sequence does not contain information about the Y chromosome. The X chromosome contains many important genes. Consequently, scientists considered it more important to obtain the high quality information for the X chromosome that was available from sequencing a female individual, as this can provide more complete information about the genes and sequence on the X chromosome. The Y chromosome could then be sequenced at a later time.

Identification of genetic variation at the DNA level for horses

One of the reasons for sequencing the whole genome was to identify genetic markers covering all of the horse chromosomes. At the beginning of the horse genome project, variation had been found for approximately 50 horse genes in connection with blood typing tests. Investigating genetic variation at the sequence level makes it easier to find variation. Firstly, there are more chances for variation when evaluating 2.43 billion DNA bp as opposed to evaluating just 20,322 proteins. Second, the techniques for studying DNA are standard, automated and inexpensive compared with the approaches for characterizing proteins.

One of the most common types of genetic variation detectable at the DNA level is called a single nucleotide polymorphism (SNP and pronounced "SNiP"). Figure 3.2

Horse 1	ATGGCTTAGGCATTTGATGGGT...
Horse 2	ATGGCTTAGGCATTTGATGGGT...
Horse 3	ATGGCTCAGGCATTTGATGGGT...
Horse 4	ATGGCTCAGGCATTTGATGGGT...
Horse 5	ATGGCTCAGGCATTTGATGGGT...

SNP= T vs C

Fig. 3.2. Comparison of base sequences of DNA strands illustrating a single nucleotide polymorphism (SNP). A hypothetical sequence is shown for five horses. The bold letter denotes the presence of a SNP, a site at which two horses have a T and three horses have a C.

illustrates a SNP. From the previous chapter, recall that DNA is made up of billions of bases called nucleotides. There are four types, abbreviated A, T, G and C. When a single one of them is mutated it may change from A to C, or G to T, or C to A, etc. When that happens, the DNA can exist in two forms at that site – essentially, it becomes polymorphic.

Twilight was the only horse completely sequenced in the horse genome project. As she has two copies of each chromosome, many SNPs were discovered just from sequencing her DNA. However, this provided limited information for genetic investigations in other horses. Therefore, DNA samples from seven other horses were sequenced at random sites in order to identify additional SNPs. These seven additional horses were chosen to represent diverse other breeds. This aspect of the project resulted in the discovery of nearly 2 million SNPs. These SNPs are identified in the online database EquCab2.0 (horse_snp_release/v2/) from the Broad Institute (see Websites section for URL). This information provides a valuable resource for scientists to investigate the genetics of horses.

Uses of Genome/DNA Variation

The techniques for investigating DNA continue to evolve. The methods used 2 years ago have been replaced. The methods we use today are likely to be eclipsed by newer, less costly approaches. Science technology moves rapidly. Scientists will use the techniques, but horse breeders need only the derived information, and do not need to become molecular geneticists. Tests have been developed, and will continue to be developed, for a wide range of traits. So far, many of the traits have been coat color genes. The genetics of coat color are well understood and breeders are interested in having such tests. The genes for coat color have also been instructive in identifying many of the different types of DNA changes that affect gene expression. These genes are discussed in greater detail in later chapters; we mention them here simply to illustrate the range of genetic variation that scientists can consider.

Changes in DNA affecting genes

Mutations changing an amino acid in a protein

These include mutations in the coat color genes *Extension* or *MC1R*, aka Black/Bay/Chestnut (Marklund *et al.*, 1996; see Chapter 4), *Cream dilution* (Mariat *et al.*, 2003;

see Chapter 5) and *Champagne dilution* (Cook *et al.*, 2008; see Chapter 5). These three coat color genes show genetic variation because of a SNP in the gene that changes an amino acid making up the protein. Changes in amino acids can alter receptor function or disable enzymatic function.

Deletion/loss of function

The Lavender Foal Syndrome (Brooks *et al.*, 2010; see Chapter 12) involves a deletion in the coding sequence for a protein which destroys the function of that protein by shifting the reading frame for translating the DNA sequence into the protein. In addition to a color variant, these foals die of multiple neurological abnormalities.

Changes in gene structure (splicing)

The *Sabino* mutation, which causes a particular pattern of white spotting (see Chapter 6), occurs between segments of a gene (exons) in one of the intron regions (Brooks and Bailey, 2005). This mutation disrupts the signal that causes the next exon to be added to the protein. In this case, although it is changed, the protein continues to operate, but has an altered function with respect to pigmentation.

Chromosome inversions

The *Tobiano* mutation, which causes white spotting (Brooks *et al.*, 2008; see Chapter 6), occurs well outside the gene that is thought to be responsible for the tobiano color pattern. In this case, the mutation is a major chromosome rearrangement; 50 megabases of DNA near the gene have an inverted order when compared with that of other horses. The precise effect of this mutation is not known but thought to affect DNA outside the gene that regulates expression of the gene.

Changes affecting gene expression

The mutation affecting the gene for appaloosa (leopard spotting) (Bellone *et al.*, 2010; see Chapter 9), like that for the *Tobiano* mutation, occurs outside the DNA coding for the gene itself. In this case, the mutation is thought to affect the signals that control when the gene is expressed.

DNA Sequencing in Horses in Addition to Twilight

The cost of whole genome sequencing has decreased dramatically during the past few years. At time of writing one of the goals for human research is to be able to sequence a mammalian genome for less than US$1000. If this becomes possible, then it may become common to sequence horses as an aid to selective breeding. The DNA sequence for an American Quarter Horse has also now been published and compared with the reference sequence reported for Twilight (Doan *et al.*, 2012a). Whole genome sequencing is becoming a routine approach for genetic studies, and hundreds of horses will have their genomes sequenced within the next few years. Why is this important?

The genome sequence of Twilight is a powerful reference for comparison with other horses. However, we are aware that differences in genome organization occur between horses. For example, we know of a major chromosome rearrangement associated with the tobiano coat color (Brooks *et al.*, 2008). We are also aware that the number of genes in the major histocompatibility complex (MHC) can vary between horses, potentially reflecting differences in immune response (Fraser and Bailey, 1998). Therefore, it was not surprising that the DNA sequence comparisons of 16 horses from 15 different breeds revealed thousands of genome rearrangements (Doan *et al.*, 2012b). The effects of these genetic differences are unknown but will be subject of further research. Twilight's genome sequence is a wonderful reference point, but we will learn more about horse genetics and genomics as we sequence more horses.

DNA Transcription/gene Expression

As noted earlier in this chapter, one of the great surprises from sequencing the genome was the discovery that most of our DNA does not code for genes. For a brief time, people jokingly referred to such DNA as junk! We just did not know what function it might serve. Since then, we have learned that almost all DNA is transcribed; that is, it is read and used to make corresponding RNA molecules. For a long time, we thought that RNA only carried out two functions in a cell: (i) to code for genes; and (ii) to serve as part of the machinery to use DNA to make proteins. Now we realize there are over 30 different types of RNA and that these carry out a wide range of functions in a cell, including the regulation of gene expression and inhibition of virus infection. We are only at the beginning of understanding this aspect of genetics, but realize that it has an impact on all areas of biology. Genetics, genomics and DNA transcription are the foundation for future understanding of everything from infectious diseases to reproduction to nutrition.

References

Bailey, E., Graves, K.T., Cothran, E.G., Reid, R., Lear, T.L. and Ennis, R.B. (1995) Synteny mapping horse microsatellite markers using a heterohybridoma panel. *Animal Genetics* 26, 177–180.

Bellone, R.B., Forsyth, G., Leeb, T., Archer, S., Sigurdsson, S., Mauceli, E., Enquensteiner, M., Bailey, E., Sandmeyer, L. and Grahn, B. (2010) Fine mapping and mutation analysis of *TRPM1*, a candidate gene for *Leopard Complex* (*LP*) spotting and congenital stationary night blindness (CNSB) in horses. *Briefings in Functional Genomics and Proteomics* 9, 193–207.

Bowling, A.T., Breen, M., Chowdhary, B.P., Hirota, K., Lear, T.L., Millon, L.V., Ponce de Leon, F.A., Raudsepp, T. and Stranzinger, G. (Committee) (1997) International system for cytogenetic nomenclature of the domestic horse. Report of the Third International Committee for the Standardization of the domestic horse karyotype, Davis, CA, USA, 1996. *Chromosome Research* 5, 443–453.

Brooks, S.A. and Bailey, E. (2005) Exon skipping in the *KIT* gene causes the sabino spotting pattern in horses. *Mammalian Genome*, 16, 893–902.

Brooks, S.A., Lear, T.L., Adelson, D.A. and Bailey, E. (2008) A chromosome inversion near the *KIT* gene and the tobiano spotting pattern in horses. *Cytogenetics and Genome Research* 119, 225–230.

Brooks, S.A., Gabreski, N., Miller, D., Brisbin, A., Brown, H.E., Streeter, C., Mezey, J., Cook, D. and Antczak, D. (2010) Whole-genome SNP association in the horse: identification of a deletion in myosin Va responsible for Lavender Foal Syndrome. *PLoS Genetics* 6(4): e1000909.

Caetano, A.R., Shiue, Y.L., Lyons, L.A., O'Brien, S.J., Laughlin, T.F., Bowling, A.T. and Murray, J.D. (1999) A comparative gene map of the horse (*Equus caballus*). *Genome Research* 9, 1239–1249.

Coleman, S.J., Zeng, Z., Wang, K., Luo, S., Khrebtukova, I., Mienaltowski, M.J., Schroth, G.P., Liu, J. and MacLeod, J.N. (2010) Structural annotation of equine protein-coding genes determined by mRNA sequencing. *Animal Genetics* 41 (Supplement 2), 121–130.

Cook, D., Brooks, S.A., Bellone, R. and Bailey, E. (2008) Missense mutation in exon 2 of SLC36A1 responsible for champagne dilution in horses. *PLoS Genetics* 4(9): e1000195.

Doan, R., Cohen, N.D., Sawyer, J., Ghaffari, N., Johnson, C.D. and Dindot, S.V. (2012a) Whole-genome sequencing and genetic variant analysis of a Quarter Horse mare. *BMC Genomics* 13: 78.

Doan, R., Cohen, N., Harrington, J., Veazy, K., Juras, R., Cothran, G., McCue, M.E., Skow, L. and Dindot, S.V. (2012b) Identification of copy number variants in horses. *Genome Research* 22, 899–907.

Fraser, D. and Bailey, E. (1998) Polymorphism and multiple loci for the horse *DQA* gene. *Immunogenetics* 47, 487–490.

International Human Genome Sequencing Consortium (2001) Initial sequencing and analysis of the human genome. *Nature* 409, 860–921.

Lear, T.L., Brandon, R., Piumi, F., Terry, R.R., Guérin, G., Thomas, S. and Bailey, E. (2001) Mapping 31 horse genes in BACs by FISH: identification of chromosomal rearrangements and conserved synteny relative to the human gene map. *Chromosome Research* 9, 261–262.

Mariat, D., Taourit, S. and Guérin, G. (2003) A mutation in the *MATP* gene causes the cream coat color in the horse. *Genetics Selection Evolution* 35, 119–133.

Marklund, L., Johansson, M.M., Sandberg, K. and Andersson, L. (1996) A missense mutation in the gene for melanocyte-stimulating hormone receptor (*MC1R*) is associated with the chestnut coat color in horses. *Mammalian Genome* 7, 895–899.

Milenkovic, D., Oustry-Vaiman, A., Lear, T., Billault, A., Mariat, D., Piumi, F., Schibler, L., Cribiu, E. and Guérin, G. (2002) Cytogenetic localization of 136 genes in the horse: comparative mapping with the human genome. *Mammalian Genome* 13, 524–534.

Penedo, M.C.T. *et al.* (2005) International Equine Gene Mapping Workshop Report: a comprehensive linkage map constructed with data from new markers and by merging four mapping resources. *Cytogenetics and Genome Research* 111, 5–15.

Raudsepp, T., Fronicke, L., Scherthan, H., Gustavsson, I. and Chowdhary, B.P. (1996) Zoo-FISH delineates conserved chromosomal segments in horse and man. *Chromosome Research* 4, 218–225.

Raudsepp, T. *et al.* (2010) A 4103 marker integrated physical and comparative map of the horse genome. *Cytogenetics and Genome Research* 122, 28–36.

Shiue, Y.-L. *et al.* (1999) A synteny map of the horse genome comprised of 240 microsatellite and RAPD markers. *Animal Genetics* 30, 1–9.

Swinburne, J.E. *et al.* (2006) Single linkage group per chromosome genetic linkage map for the horse, based on two three-generation, full-sibling, crossbred horse reference families. *Genomics* 87, 1–29.

Venter, J.C. *et al.* (2001) The sequence of the human genome. *Science* 291, 1304–1351.

Wade, C.M. *et al.* (2009) Genome sequence, comparative analysis and population genetics of the domestic horse (*Equus caballus*). *Science* 326, 865–867.

Websites

Broad Institute of Harvard and MIT (Massachusetts Institute of Technology), Massachusetts. Horse Genome Project. Available at: http://www.broadinstitute.org/mammals/horse (accessed 10 December 2012); horse SNPs available at online database EquCab2.0 (horse_snp_release/v2/) from the Broad Institute Horse Genome Project: http://www.broadinstitute.org/ftp/distribution/horse_snp_release/v2/ (accessed 1 January 2013).

ENSEMBL project, Cambridge, UK. Available at: http://uswest.ensembl.org/Equus_caballus/Info/Index (accessed 10 December 2012).

Genome Center at University of California at Santa Cruz. Available at: http://www.genome.ucsc.edu (accessed 10 December 2012).

Horse Genome Project, Coordinator Dr Ernest Bailey, Gluck Equine Research Center, Department of Veterinary Science, University of Kentucky, Lexington, Kentucky. Available at: http://www.uky.edu/Ag/Horsemap (accessed 13 December 2012).

National Center for Biological Information (NCBI), Washington, DC. Available at: http://www.ncbi.nlm.nih.gov/mapview/map_search.cgi?taxid=9796 (accessed 10 December 2012).

National Human Genome Research Institute (NHGRI), Bethesda, Maryland. Available at: http://www.genome.gov/ (accessed 14 December 2012).

4 Black, Bay, and Chestnut (*Extension* and *Agouti*)

It is likely that the ancestral color of the horse was a black-based pattern that provided camouflage protection against predators. The coat might have resembled that of the modern-day Przewalski's horse, the surviving wild species most closely related to domestic horses, which is typically described as dun. Regardless of the true ancestral color, under domestication the horse has clearly evolved into an animal with a wide range of coat variation. In fact, research using DNA-based tests for coat color alleles has been used with ancient DNA samples to assess the color of prehistoric horses. This work demonstrated that many of the modern colors and spotting patterns that we observe today were very rapidly acquired by the horse around 5000 years ago, very shortly after domestication (Ludwig *et al.*, 2009).

The different color patterns are controlled by genetic differences that occurred initially as random mutations and have since been selected for during the course of domestication. In mammals, melanin is the most important pigment of coat color. It occurs as pigment granules in the hair, skin, and iris as well as in some internal tissues. Melanin is made in two related forms: eumelanin (black or brown) and pheomelanin (red or yellow) (Searle, 1968). The biochemistry of pigment production in the horse is homologous to that of other species (Woolf and Swafford, 1988). Genes produce coat color variation by altering the switch between eumelanin and pheomelanin production in pigment cells (melanocytes), or by the presence, shape, number, or arrangement of pigment granules. Color names for many phenotypes are easy to designate by visual inspection. Owners and breed registries often record colors as one means of identifying individuals. This word description of the color phenotype can suggest which alleles a particular animals might possess for pigment synthesis and distribution. However, there are several key limitations of word descriptions:

- Most breeds have a rather restricted set of recognized color names compared with the variation of hues that exists. Although frustrating at times, this may be an appropriate policy because much of the variation in shade and intensity within colors is not yet defined by adequate genetic models.
- Two breeds may use different names for colors that appear to be the same, or the same name for colors that are genetically different.
- Phenotypic descriptions can provide an approximation of the genes involved and a working model to predict the color outcome of different matings. It should be emphasized though that two horses with the same word description may not have the same genotype.
- DNA-based tests for the color genes of the horse most reliably describe the alleles carried by an individual, and therefore the potential to pass these alleles on to offspring.

The *Extension* locus (*E*) is responsible for the base coat color of horses. Other genes, including *Agouti* (*A*), act to modify or mask the effects of the *Extension* locus. Together, *Extension* and *Agouti* are responsible for the most common color patterns of horses, namely, black, bay and chestnut (red). Plate 1 shows Thoroughbred and draft cross mares exemplifying the chestnut (left) and bay (right) base coat colors. Near the turn of the 19th century, Hurst (1906) showed that Thoroughbred stud book color records could be explained using genes inherited according to Mendelian principles.

Extension

In the horse, the *Extension* locus is credited with producing the black pigment (eumelanin) observed in blacks, browns, bays, buckskins, duns and grullas, as well as the red pigment (pheomelanin) seen in chestnuts, sorrels, palominos and red duns. Initially, this locus was called *Brown* (*B*) but the *Extension* locus terminology became preferred as it was clearly the same as the *Extension* genes already identified in other mammals.

Trait inheritance and gene symbol

Two alleles of extension are assigned to account for the black/chestnut color variation in horses. The alleles either extend (*E*) or diminish (*e*) the amount of eumelanin (black) in the coat, thus exerting the opposite effect on the visible extent of pheomelanin (red). In the simplest terms, the extension gene determines whether black pigment is found in the hair and skin (*EE* or *Ee*), or only in the skin (*ee*) (see Table 4.1).

A second and important aspect of black hair pigment in horses is its distribution. Black hair may be distributed uniformly across the body, as found in a black horse, or in a pattern called bay where it is restricted to the mane, tail and legs but reduced or absent on the body. Black pattern characteristics are due to a second gene (*Agouti* aka *ASIP*), which is discussed in the next section of this chapter.

The presence of black pigment is inherited as a trait dominant (*E*) to its absence (*e*), so matings between two chestnut (*ee*) horses will not produce any black/brown/bay offspring. This "chestnut rule" has been repeatedly verified by parentage exclusion in exceptional cases (Trommershausen-Smith *et al.*, 1976).

The intensity of pigmentation can vary for both chestnut and black horses. Some chestnut horses have very light, red coats, sometimes called "light sorrel", while others exhibit a much darker coloration and are often called "liver chestnut". Likewise, horses that are genetically black can show graded variation in color such

Table 4.1. Genotypes and phenotypes for the *Extension* (*E*) allele.

Color	Genotype
Black, brown or bay	*EE* or *Ee*
Chestnut (red)	*ee*

that the visual impact of some black horses is to appear as brown. The *Extension* locus is not responsible for this type of variation. Other, as yet unknown, modifying loci are likely responsible for this variation in intensity. Other variants that can appear include "Bend D'Or" spots, which are small, irregular dark hair patches found on chestnut horses that look like black smudges on the red coat. Similarly, small white patches in the coat are known as "Birdcatcher" spots. Eumelanin production in the hair appears to break through in these *ee* horses, but not to such an extent that they could be confused with *E–* horses.

Molecular genetics and gene location

The *Extension* gene, *E*, is also termed the *MC1R* gene. Initial mapping of the *MC1R* gene located it on ECA3 along with another important color gene, *KIT* (Raudsepp *et al.*, 1999; see Chapter 6). According to the second assembly of the horse genome sequence (EquCab2), *MC1R* can be found at chr3:36259305-36260257.

The genetic change responsible for the mutation of the *E* allele to the *e* allele was a missense mutation of a single nucleotide in the *Melanocortin 1 Receptor* gene (*MC1R*) (Marklund *et al.*, 1996). This alteration of the genetic code results in the substitution of a phenylalanine for a serine in a portion of the protein that crosses the cell membrane. This change destroys the receptor function of the *MC1R* molecule that results in the production of eumelanin. Therefore, horses homozygous for this mutation cannot produce black pigment … with the unexplained exceptions of Bend D'Or spots and other minor exceptions mentioned above.

A third, very rare allele of *MC1R* has been found for chestnut color. This allele, designated *ea*, is functionally equivalent to the *e* allele but interferes with its detection in many standard DNA tests (Wagner and Reissmann, 2000). Horses with this allele possess the mutation responsible for *e* plus a second mutation, very nearby, that interferes with detection of *e* when using some testing methods. While this mutation changes the DNA, it does not change the protein. Therefore, breeders will only become aware of this allele when they obtain test results inconsistent with the color of the horse: specifically, chestnut horses reported to possess the *E* allele by the DNA test laboratory.

A fourth allele of *MC1R* in horses (called E^D, though as noted in Chapter 2 we would advocate the use of *ED* for this name) has been proposed to account for "dominant black"; however, the genetic basis for this allele has yet to be discovered (Rieder *et al.*, 2001).

Gene function

MC1R was a good candidate for *Extension* in horses because it was known to have several alleles that affect black hair distribution in mice. In fact, a eumelanin/pheomelanin switch is seen in the hair colors of many mammalian species and is a prominent source of color variation among domestic animals. Labrador Retriever dogs may be black or yellow (or chocolate, but that is a gene story we will not be discussing in the horse context). Holstein and Angus are predominantly black-pigmented cattle breeds, but red animals occur and some owners specifically select for the red color. In both examples, alleles of the *MC1R* gene have been identified as controlling red/black base coat colors.

From studies in mice, it is known that *MC1R* codes for a receptor protein that is part of the membrane of melanocytes, the cells that make pigment. Once this receptor binds its specific signaling hormone (melanocyte stimulating hormone) it triggers the cell to make eumelanin (black pigment). Recessive alleles of *MC1R* in the mouse fail to bind the melanocyte stimulating hormone, so only pheomelanin, and not eumelanin, is made (Robbins *et al.*, 1993). Other alleles cause the receptor to bind the hormone so tightly that eumelanin is always made.

MC1R also plays a role in some other signaling pathways. In the brain, for example, it has been shown to be important in the perception of pain. Studies of people with red hair, as a result of a human *MC1R* allele, have shown that they are more sensitive to pain, and receive less relief from certain analgesic drugs (Mogil *et al.*, 2005). Given the similarities in the type of mutation, this same effect may be present in chestnut horses, although this remains to be investigated.

Breeds

Most horse breeds include both red- and black-pigmented variants, but a few breeds have little or no variation for this gene. Friesians and Cleveland Bays have only the dominant allele of *Extension*, E. Rare recessives could be present but are extremely difficult to detect without the use of a DNA-based test. In contrast, Suffolks and Haflingers have only the recessive allele of *Extension*, e.

Agouti

Bay horses have a deep red body with black mane, tail, and lower limbs. The body shade varies from a bright "blood bay" to a deeper "mahogany bay". Bay horses are more common than black or chestnut horses among Thoroughbred and Standardbred horses. The coat of black horses can vary in hue and have a uniform distribution of black pigment throughout the hair coat (see Plate 2).

Trait inheritance and gene symbol

The dominant allele *A* of the *Agouti* gene causes the distribution of eumelanin in hair to be restricted to a "points" pattern (e.g. mane, tail, ear rims, lower legs) (see Plate 1). The recessive allele *a* does not restrict the distribution of black hair, and when homozygous in the presence of *E*, it produces a uniformly black horse (see Table 4.2).

Breeders specializing in black horses will want to understand the special combination of the two genes *Extension* and *Agouti* that are required to obtain the desired color. Predicting whether given matings will produce black is complicated by the uncertainty about which *Agouti* alleles are present in chestnut (*ee*) horses. In many breeds, the *a* allele is rare (black horses are infrequent), so most bays and chestnuts

Table 4.2. Phenotypes for combinations of the *E* and *A* alleles.

Phenotype	Genotype
Bay or brown	*EEAA, EeAA, EEAa,* or *EeAa*
Black	*EEaa* or *Eeaa*
Chestnut (red)	*eeAA, eeAa,* or *eeaa*

are *AA*. Any red or bay horse that sires or produces a black offspring must be carrying *a*. If a chestnut horse has two black (*Eeaa*) parents then he must be *eeaa*.

Black coat color varies from blue-black to sun-fading black, but the genetic differences among the variations are currently undefined. Other alleles hypothesized for agouti in horses (described as *A+ or A'* in earlier studies) have been proposed to define the inheritance of wild pattern (as in Przewalski's horse) and brown horses, but they have not been studied extensively. Alternative alleles of *Agouti* might be responsible for some of the variation in pigment distribution of color shades of bays, seal browns, and blacks.

Molecular genetics and gene location

The *Agouti signaling peptide* gene (*ASIP*) has been identified as the cause of *Agouti* (*A*) in horses (Rieder *et al.*, 2001). *ASIP* controls the distribution pattern of eumelanin, so its actions are obvious only in the presence of *E* (an example of epistatic gene interaction). The *Agouti* gene is located on ECA22 at chr22:25,167,080-25,171,073 in the EquCab2 assembly of the genome. The *a* allele results from the deletion of 11 nucleotides from the sequence for the *ASIP* gene (Rieder *et al.*, 2001). It is thought that loss of these nucleotides destroys the function of the peptide. Additional alleles of *ASIP* have been proposed (*At*, responsible for seal brown or black and tan; and *A+*, wild bay) but results of these studies have not yet been published and the genetic basis for these alleles is not widely known. Testing for the *a* allele is available at several laboratories and is often coupled with the test for the *MC1R* alleles in order to predict the base color of offspring.

Gene function

The gene derives its name from a South American rodent with black-banded hairs. In the dog, four *Agouti* alleles are known, including recessive black, black and tan, wild type and fawn (Schmutz and Berryere, 2007). Several alleles are also observed in cattle, including recessive black, lighter points and a regulatory mutation leading to a brindle pattern (Girardot *et al.*, 2006; Seo *et al.*, 2007). The agouti signaling peptide regulates the production of eumelanin versus pheomelanin synthesis, either during hair growth phases (black-banded yellow hairs) or spatially (black hairs on the back, but not on the abdomen). It competes with melanocyte stimulating hormone for binding to *MC1R*, thus affected the cellular "switch" for pigment type. This signaling system is also important in the control of fat storage in adipocytes. Several mouse alleles of *ASIP* result not only in coat color variation but also in obesity.

Breeds

The uniformly bay Cleveland Bay breed has only the *A* allele; black horses are never produced. Friesians are all black and therefore have only the *a* allele for *Agouti*. The distribution of black versus bay horses in a population depends on the frequency of alleles for this gene. Most light horse breeds appear to have a higher frequency of *A* than *a* (and therefore are bay), but for pony and draft breeds with a high prevalence of chestnut horses, the frequency relationship may be reversed with an increase of black horses.

References

Girardot, M., Guibert, S., Laforet, M.P., Gallard, Y., Larroque, H. and Oulmouden, A. (2006) The insertion of a full-length *Bos taurus* LINE element is responsible for a transcriptional deregulation of the Normande *Agouti* gene. *Pigment Cell Research* 19, 346–355.

Hurst, C.C. (1906) On the inheritance of coat colour in horses. *Proceedings of the Royal Society, Series B* 77, 388–394.

Ludwig, A., Pruvost, M., Reissmann, M., Benecke, N., Brockmann, G.A., Castanos, P., Cieslak, M., Lippold, S., Llorente, L., Malaspinas, A.S., Slatkin, M. and Hofreiter, M. (2009) Coat color variation at the beginning of horse domestication. *Science* 324, 485.

Marklund, L., Moller, M.J., Sandberg, K. and Andersson, L. (1996) A missense mutation in the gene for melanocyte-stimulating hormone receptor (*MC1R*) is associated with the chestnut coat color in horses. *Mammalian Genome* 7, 895–899.

Mogil, J.S., Ritchie, J., Smith, S.B., Strasburg, K., Kaplan, L., Wallace, M.R., Romberg, R.R., Bijl, H., Sarton, E.Y., Fillingim, R.B. and Dahan, A. (2005) Melanocortin-1 receptor gene variants affect pain and µ-opioid analgesia in mice and humans. *Journal of Medical Genetics* 42, 583–587.

Raudsepp, T., Kijas, J., Godard, S., Guerin, G., Andersson, L. and Chowdhary, B.P. (1999) Comparison of horse chromosome 3 with donkey and human chromosomes by cross-species painting and heterologous FISH mapping. *Mammalian Genome* 10, 277–282.

Rieder, S., Taourit, S., Mariat, D., Langlois, B. and Guérin, G. (2001) Mutations in the agouti (*ASIP*), the extension (*MC1R*), and the brown (*TYRP1*) loci and their association to coat color phenotypes in horses (*Equus caballus*). *Mammalian Genome* 12, 450–455.

Robbins, L.S., Nadeau, J.H., Johnson, K.R., Kelly, M.A., Roselli-Rehfuss, L., Baack, E., Mountjoy, K.G. and Cone, R.D. (1993) Pigmentation phenotypes of variant extension locus alleles result from point mutations that alter MSH receptor function. *Cell* 72, 827–834.

Schmutz, S.M. and Berryere, T.G. (2007) Genes affecting coat colour and pattern in domestic dogs: a review. *Animal Genetics* 38, 539–549.

Searle, A.G. (1968) *Comparative Genetics of Coat Colour in Mammals*. Logos Press, London/New York.

Seo, K., Mohanty, T.R., Choi, T. and Hwang, I. (2007) Biology of epidermal and hair pigmentation in cattle: a mini-review. *Veterinary Dermatology* 18, 392–400.

Trommershausen-Smith, A., Suzuki, Y. and Stormont, C. (1976) Use of blood typing to confirm principles of coat-color genetics in horses. *Journal of Heredity* 67, 6–10.

Wagner, H.J. and Reissmann, M. (2000) New polymorphism detected in the horse *MC1R* gene. *Animal Genetics* 31, 289–290.

Woolf, C.M. and Swafford, J.R. (1988) Evidence for eumelanin and pheomelanin producing genotypes in the Arabian horse. *Journal of Heredity,* 79, 100–106.

5   Color Diluting Genes

Coat color dilution in horses is due to the actions of at least four genes, *Cream* (*C*), *Dun* (*D*), *Silver* (*Z*) and *Champagne* (*CH*). These genes dilute the black (eumelanin) and red (pheomelanin) pigments produced as a consequence of gene action by the *Extension* locus (*E* or *MC1R*) modified by the *Agouti* (*A*) locus; see Chapter 4. As the effect of the dilution genes is to modify the action of another locus (*E*), the dilution genes are described as having an epistatic effect on coat color. These genes are well known to horse owners and popular for many breeds. Molecular genetic studies have led to the discoveries of the genes and the DNA mutations responsible for three of these four dilution genes.

Cream Dilution

The most widely recognized of the color dilution genes is the one that produces the golden body color seen in palominos (Plate 3) and buckskins (Plate 4). A palomino horse has a white (flaxen) mane and tail while a buckskin has black mane, tail, and legs. The *Cream Dilution* gene reduces the intensity of the red pigment (pheomelanin) and modestly reduces the intensity of the black pigment. Diluting the red hair of chestnuts produces a palomino pattern, while dilution of the red hair for bays produces a buckskin pattern.

The skin and eyes of palominos and buckskins are dark, although they may be lighter than those of non-diluted colors. Sometimes, the mane and tail of the palomino or the body color of the buckskin have dark hairs intermixed, reflecting the similar admixtures found in the undiluted dark bay or chestnut counterparts. Palominos can be very light cream when born. A darker golden color becomes obvious after the foal coat is shed. Buckskins may also be light when born, even to a degree that the black points may not be obvious until the foal is some weeks old. These colors may also vary seasonally, being lighter in the winter coat.

Cremellos are "double dilutes" based on chestnuts with two copies of the *Cream Dilution* gene, while perlinos are double dilutes of bays with two copies of the *Cream Dilution* gene. Cremellos have pink skin, blue eyes and ivory hair. Perlinos have the same features, except that the mane and tail are slightly darker than the body.

As described in Chapter 4, it is not obvious that black horses (*aaE–*) have red pigment. However, one or two copies of the *Cream Dilution* gene exhibit moderate dilution effects on these horses, producing a phenotype sometimes described as "smokey".

A third allele has been identified for the *Cream Dilution* locus, which is called the *Pearl Dilution*. This allele interacts with the *Cream Dilution* gene to produce coat color dilutions that are very similar to the Champagne Dilution phenotypes described below.

Trait inheritance and gene symbol

The gene symbol used for the *Cream Dilution* locus is C. This gene symbol was first used in other mammals to denote the locus for albinism and was subsequently used to describe horses that had white or near white coats (Castle, 1948). Even though actual albino horses are exceptionally rare, this terminology has continued to be used for *Cream Dilution* (Bowling, 1996; Sponenberg, 2009). Because this locus has nothing to do with albinism, it would be appropriate for a body of scientists to rename the locus symbol as "CR" for *Cream Dilution*. But for the time being we will continue to refer to it as the C locus.

The C locus has three known alleles. The gene causing the dilution effect is an incomplete dominant and we use the symbol "CR" to designate that allele. The absence of dilution is recessive and the symbolic representation we use for this allele is "cr". As noted above, a third allele has also been reported for this locus, called *Pearl*. This allele is reported to have a recessive mode of inheritance and we use the symbol "prl" to identify it.

Genetics of *CR* and *cr* in bay, chestnut and black horses

The action of CR is to dilute pheomelanin (red) to yellow when heterozygous, while having little effect on eumelanin (black). Both eumelanin and pheomelanin are diluted to pale ivory when the dilution allele is homozygous *(CRCR)* (Adalsteinsson, 1974); see Table 5.1.

When we combine the dilution gene symbols with those for the coat color genes involved with the basic production of color, palominos are diluted reds *(CRcr ee)* and buckskins are diluted bays *(A–E– CRcr)*. Blacks *(aaE– CRcr)*, can carry the dilution gene without expressing it, because they do not have visible red pigment to show the single dose effects of the dilution gene. Sometimes, the presence of the dilution gene in black horses may not be recognized and breeders will be surprised when a palomino or buckskin offspring is produced from breeding a non-diluted horse *(crcr)* to a black horse. Molecular testing can verify the situation.

Why the palomino has a white mane and tail, not gold like the body color, is not easily explained, but could be related to differences in gene action between the mel-

Table 5.1. Genotypes and phenotypes for the *CR* allele of the *Cream Dilution* (C) locus; *cr* denotes the absence of dilution and is recessive.

Phenotype	Genotype
Not dilute	*crcr*
Palomino/buckskin	*CRcr*
Cremello/perlino	*CRCR*

anocytes (pigment producing cells) of the permanent hair (mane and tail) compared with those of the seasonally shed hair.

Novice breeders, captivated by the beauty of the palomino and buckskin colors, are discouraged to learn that neither will breed true as the desirable colors are produced by heterozygosity for a dilution gene. If a breeder attempts to duplicate the color of a favorite palomino, say by breeding that palomino to another palomino, the predicted colors and their frequencies among the offspring will be 50% palomino, 25% chestnut and 25% cremello (see Table 5.2). For some breeds, a cremello (or perlino) is undesirable, or even cannot be registered. In this case, the better mating choice would be palomino × chestnut; the expected proportion of palominos for this cross is the same as that from a palomino × palomino mating (50%) but no cremellos would be anticipated. In breeds that allow the registration of cremello and perlino – colors such as Icelandic, Miniature, Peruvian Paso, or Paso Fino – a homozygous diluted horse can be an important component for a breeding program specializing in palominos and buckskins. The cremello or perlino will contribute a color dilution gene to all offspring, resulting in the desired heterozygous genotype when mated to non-diluted individuals (Plate 5).

Genetics of the *Pearl (prl)* allele

The *Pearl Dilution* allele (*prl*) has been described in review by Sponenberg (2009). *Pearl Dilution* is a recessive allele and horses with a single copy of the *Pearl Dilution* allele and the non-dilute allele (genotype: *crprl*) do not exhibit dilution and will appear as bay, chestnut, or black. However, in the presence of *CR*, e.g. in the genotype *CRprl*, the effect of the dilution approaches the appearance of horses with a copy of the *Cream Dilution* gene and a copy of the *Champagne Dilution* gene (*CRcr* and *CHch*), which produces greater dilution of the pheomelanin and a modest dilution of eumelanin. (The *Champagne* gene is described in the last section of this chapter.) For a horse with two copies of *prl*, the effect is nearly identical to the colors produced by heterozygotes for *Champagne*, but defined to reflect the different genetic origin: chestnut becomes pearl gold, bay becomes amber or sable pearl, and black becomes classic pearl.

The effects of each possible genotype for the *Cream Dilution* locus on the base coat colors are shown in Table 5.3.

Table 5.2. Punnett square for mating a palomino mare (*ee CRcr*) and stallion (*ee CRcr*). Palominos will only be produced 2 in 4 times, cremellos 1 in 4 times, and chestnuts 1 in 4 times.

Genetic contribution from mare eggs (*ee CRcr*)	Genetic contribution from stallion sperm (*ee CRcr*)	
	e CR	*e cr*
e CR	*ee CRCR*	*ee CRcr*
Color of cross	Cremello	Palomino
e cr	*ee CRcr*	*ee crcr*
Color of cross	Palomino	Chestnut

Table 5.3. Genotypes and phenotypes for alleles of the *Cream Dilution* locus (*C*) with different base color phenotypes.

Base color phenotype and genotype (*A, E* loci)	*C* genotype	Phenotypic effect
Chestnut (– – *ee*)	*crcr*	Chestnut
	CRcr	Palomino
	CRCR	Cremello
	crprl	Chestnut
	CRprl	Nearly white
	prlprl	Gold pearl
Bay (*A– E–*)	*crcr*	Bay
	CRcr	Buckskin
	CRCR	Perlino
	crprl	Bay
	CRprl	Beige, brown points
	prlprl	Amber pearl
Black (*aa E–*)	*crcr*	Black
	CRcr	Black (smokey?)
	CRCR	Smoky cream
	crprl	Black
	CRprl	Tan, tan points
	prlprl	Classic pearl

Molecular genetics and gene location

The locus of the *CR* allele was initially mapped to ECA21 using microsatellites (see Chapter 11) and family studies (Locke *et al.*, 2001). Later, *CR* was shown to be an allele of *SLC45A2* (solute carrier family 45, member 2 gene, previously known as *MATP*, the gene for the membrane associated transport protein) (Mariat *et al.*, 2003). *SLC45A2* is located at chr21:30,664,390-30,693,166 in the EquCab2 genome assembly. A missense mutation in the second exon of *SLC45A2* results in the exchange of an aspartic acid for an asparagine in the amino acid sequence. This polymorphism is easily detected and a genetic test for it is widely available.

Gene function

Polymorphisms of the *SLC45A2* gene result in variations in human skin, hair and eye color, from dark to fair. More severe mutations result in oculocutaneous albinism type IV. In the mouse, variations at the locus result in dilution of the under-fur, skin, and eyes. This gene is also responsible for a form of albinism and silver feather color in the chicken. Although it has also been investigated as a candidate gene for cream color in dogs, no association has yet been made (Schmutz and Berryere, 2007).

The function of *SLC45A2* is not completely understood, though it is known to mediate the synthesis of melanin thorough transport of the tyrosinase enzyme (Costin *et al.*, 2003).

Breeds

The *CR* allele occurs in a variety of breeds. It is typically associated with ponies and stock horse breeds, but also occurs in Paso Finos, Peruvian Pasos, American Saddlebreds, Morgans and Tennessee Walking horses. Palominos and buckskins occur among US Thoroughbreds, but they are very rare. This dilution gene is probably absent from Arabians. While Arabian iridescent light chestnuts with extremely flaxen manes and tails may be registered with palomino societies, the buckskin and cremello counterpart colors to palomino are not seen in this breed.

The *Pearl* allele has been reported among Lusitano, Gypsy Cob/Vanner, and Paint horses, and among American Quarter Horses (Sponenberg, 2009). In Quarter Horses and Paints it has been referred to as the "BarLink Factor", but this has been found to be genetically identical to the factor previously described as *Pearl* (UC Davis Veterinary Medicine website; see Websites section for URL).

Health concerns

The blue eyes of cremellos and perlinos are sensitive to the sun and owners report that these horses actively seek protective shade in summer (i.e. they exhibit photophobia). Pink-skinned horses are more subject to sunburn neoplastic conditions such as squamous cell and basal cell carcinomas about the eyes (Knottenbelt and Pascoe, 1994).

Dun

In an otherwise red horse, the *Dun* gene produces a pinkish-red horse with darker red points and the complex pattern of dorsal stripe, shoulder stripe and leg bars (these three patterns are often collectively referred as "primitive markings"). This color is known as red dun or claybank dun. In a horse with a bay base coat, *Dun* produces a more or less yellow-red animal with black points and primitive markings which is known simply as dun (Plate 6). Grulla describes an otherwise black animal with the *Dun* gene which appears as a mouse-gray color with primitive markings.

Trait inheritance and gene symbol

The dominantly inherited *Dun* allele, "*D*", dilutes both the eumelanin and the pheomelanin of body hair, but does not dilute either pigment in hair on the points. The recessive alternative (not dun) is designated "*d*". The red body color is diluted to pale red (claybank or red dun) or yellow red (buckskin dun); black body hair is diluted to mouse gray (grulla) (Van Vleck and Davitt, 1977). In addition to pigment dilution, *D* is characterized as producing a coat pattern that includes a dark head, dark points, dorsal stripe, shoulder stripes, and leg bars, even though these markings may be subtle and easily go unnoticed. Among some Przewalski's horses and Mongolian ponies, the dun markings on the shoulder and upper leg may be in the form of a distinctive network or webbing pattern. Homozygotes for *D* are phenotypically indistinguishable from heterozygotes and do not show the extreme color dilution effects associated with homozygotes for the palomino/buckskin gene. Gremmel (1939) showed that in the hair shafts of duns, pigment granules are heavily concentrated on one side rather than being uniformly distributed around the core. The *D* gene may affect the clumping of pigment granules, thus providing an optical dilution effect, in contrast to the *CR* allele, which controls pigment quantity.

The allelic effects of *D* can be confused with those of *CR*, although there are several important differences. Firstly, unlike *CR*, *D* dilutes both the black and red pigment on the body but does not dilute either pigment on the points. Red body color is diluted to a pinkish red, yellowish red or yellow; black body color is diluted to mouse gray. Second, in addition to pigment dilution, a key characteristic of *D* is the striping pattern. Finally, homozygosity for *D* does not produce extreme color dilution (see Table 5.4).

A horse may have both the *CR* and *D* dilution alleles. A red horse with both dilution genes looks like a palomino with dun markings. Heterozygosity for dilution genes at both loci does not result in extreme color dilution. More or less faint primitive markings can sometimes be found on otherwise "ordinary" undiluted chestnuts and bays, and may be prominent on young grays. These dun markings without color dilution are probably the effects of another gene, but at times could be confused with those of the *D* gene.

Molecular genetics and gene location

The location of the *Dun* gene has not yet been reported. However, a genetic test is commercially available from the Veterinary Genetics Laboratory (VGL) at the University of California Davis (see UC Davis Veterinary Medicine in Websites section), based on preliminary results from research at VGL.

Gene function

Dun does not have obvious counterparts in other species. In other mammals (Searle, 1968), *d* is the symbol for dilute, a recessively inherited color gene that effects a distinctive clumping of pigment granules that produces the optical effect of color dilution. The dun color of Dexter cattle is an allele of the *TYRP1* gene, as is brown in dogs, but as polymorphisms in this gene specifically change the color of eumelanin from black to brown, this is not a candidate for dun in the horse.

Table 5.4. Genotypes and phenotypes for the *D* locus.

Phenotype	Genotype
Dun	*DD* or *Dd*
Not dun	*dd*

Breeds

In North America, the *D* allele is seen in stock horses, in ponies, and among feral horses. A prominent breed with dun is the Norwegian Fjord. The dun trait is generally found in breeds that also have *CR*, so it is important to be able to distinguish the variants of these genes both alone and in combination.

Silver Dilution

The color diluting gene *Silver Dilution*, "*Z*", is a complement to the *Cream Dilution* gene. Just as the *Cream Dilution* gene affects the red pigment with minimal effect on black pigment, the *Silver Dilution* gene dilutes black pigment. *Silver Dilution* was first described by Castle and Smith (1953) and is purported to have originated in the late 1800s among Shetland ponies. This origin was initially accepted, but the occurrence of *Silver Dilution* among horses as well as ponies suggests that it may be have an ancient origin. The color variant is sometimes called silver dapple or taffy.

The effects of the *Silver Dilution* gene are seen conspicuously on black horses (*aa E*–) in which the coat color is diluted to a chocolate or black chocolate, often with dapples, and the mane and tail are diluted to silver gray or flaxen (Plate 7). On genetically bay horses, the gene produces color dilution so that the horse is usually described as a silver-maned chestnut, but the legs retain some darker pigment. A possible color name for a bay with the silver dapple dilution is silver bay. The gene has little effect on chestnut (pheomelanin) coat color, beyond producing a slightly lighter mane and tail. This color is sometimes called silver sorrel, but it is difficult to distinguish visually from sorrel.

The addition of the word "dapple" to the name of this dilution gene is unfortunate. The name implies that dapples are always associated with this color, which is emphatically not true. The word "dapple" leads some owners to confuse this color with gray. In Miniature horses, many silver dapple horses are registered as dapple gray. Classic silver foals are born a light reddish brown color with the same color mane and tail. As the foal coat is shed, the mane and tail grow in light, and the body color darkens to deep chocolate. Silver dapple interacts with gray so that the birth color of foals with the gray allele (*G*; see Chapter 7) is comparable to that of a mature gray.

Trait inheritance and gene symbol

The silver trait is inherited as dominant, but the gene action in combination with variants at other coat color genes is poorly documented. Castle and Smith (1953) initially proposed *S* for the gene symbol, reflecting the name silver given to the color in horses, but this symbol was not suitable as it is used for spotting traits in other mammals. Currently, *Z* is used as the gene symbol for silver dapple, with *Z* and *z*, respectively, representing the dominant and recessive alleles for the presence and absence of the silver dilution trait.

As described above, this gene has no or minimal effects on chestnut horses, which are devoid of black pigment. However, a single copy of *Z* produces the dilution effects. Horses homozygous for *Z* may exhibit greater dilution, but the effect is modest. Table 5.5 shows the effects of *Z* genotypes on the base coat colors.

Table 5.5. Genotypes and phenotypes for alleles of the *Silver Dilution* gene (*Z*) with different base color phenotypes.

Base color phenotype (*A*, *E* loci)	*Z* genotype	Phenotypic effect
Chestnut (– –, *ee*)	zz	Chestnut
	Zz	Chestnut
	ZZ	Chestnut
Bay (*A–*, *E–*)	zz	Bay
	Zz	Silver mane
	ZZ	Silver mane
Black (*aa*, E–)	zz	Black
	Zz	Silver body
	ZZ	Silver body

An apparent exception to the "chestnut coat color rule" may be a consequence of the *Silver Dilution* gene (Trommershausen-Smith *et al.*, 1976). A bay horse (*A–E–*) with a dilution of the black pigment could be misidentified as a chestnut. When this silver bay (registered as a chestnut) is bred to a chestnut, offspring receiving *E*, but not the dilution gene, could be, legitimately, bay or black.

Molecular genetics and gene location

Silver is attributed to a missense mutation in the *SILV* (aka *PMEL17*) silver homolog gene (Brunberg *et al.*, 2006). The missense mutation occurs in exon 11 and results in an amino acid substitution of an arginine for a cysteine. *SILV* encodes a protein that is found on the surface of the melanosome, the pigment producing organelle in melanocytes. Its function is not fully understood, but it may play a role in the organization of melanosomes. *SILV* is located at chr6:73,665,135-73,672,980 in the EquCab2 genome assembly.

Gene function

The identical mutation of *SILV* has not been observed in other species, though other mutations in *SILV* in other species have affected coat colors. In the mouse, mutations of the *SILV* gene result in a variety of diluted colors and roan-like phenotypes. The diluted coat of Charolais cattle is also attributed to a polymorphism in *SILV* (Gutiérrez-Gil *et al.*, 2007). In contrast, the strikingly spotted coat of merle dogs is also a result of the *SILV* locus, although in this case the polymorphism is the insertion of a repeat element rather than a change in the coding sequence (Clark *et al.*, 2006).

Breeds

The silver color dilution gene is most conspicuously found in Shetland, American Miniature, and Rocky Mountain horses, and in Icelandic breeds, and but is also observed in Quarter Horses, Paints, Morgans, American Saddlebreds, and Peruvian Pasos.

Health concerns

The Multiple Congenital Ocular Anomalies (MCOA) syndrome results in a collection of eye problems, including cysts and cataracts. MCOA has been mapped to the same genetic region as *SILV* (Andersson *et al.*, 2008), and is inherited in a codominant manner. As such, homozygotes are more severely affected than heterozygotes. While many silver horses also have MCOA, the association is not complete. Some silver horses do not exhibit MCOA, and MCOA also occurs in some horses without silver. Nevertheless, this association has been strong, and it may be due to the close proximity (linkage) of two separate mutations.

Champagne Dilution

The *Champagne Dilution* (*CH*) gene is thought to be the result of a fairly recent mutation because it occurs only among horse breeds developed in North America. The *Champagne Dilution* gene is distinct from the *Cream Dilution* and *Silver Dilution* genes in that it dilutes both eumelanin and pheomelanin. On a chestnut (*ee*) base coat, the champagne dilution results in a gold body color with a light flaxen mane and tail. Gold champagnes in particular, but occasionally the other champagne shades as well, can possess an attractive metallic sheen. When present in combination with a bay base coat, champagne results in a slightly darker golden body with a dark chocolate color to the mane and tail. Hairs along the margins of the mane and tail may be even further diluted to a color more similar to the body. This combination of champagne and bay is called "amber". The "classic" champagne is a result of the champagne dilution on a black base coat. Classic champagnes have a deeper bronze body coat color and a dark chocolate mane and tail (Plate 8).

The champagne colors of gold, amber, and classic look similar to, and can be easily confused with, palomino, buckskin resulting from *CR*, and dun and grulla due to *D*. However, the colours can be uniquely distinguished by possession of lightly pigmented "pumpkin" colored skin, mottled freckling of the hairless skin, and lightened eye color, which are not commonly seen in horses possessing *cr*. Identification of the champagne dilution can be further complicated by interactions with many other color loci. Age can also alter the color, as *CH* foals are usually born with blue eyes and pink skin, which will darken somewhat with age.

Trait inheritance and gene symbol

Champagne Dilution is inherited in a dominant manner with alleles *CH* (dominant) and *ch* (recessive), so that there are few phenotypic differences between heterozygous and homozygous individuals. It can occur in combination with the other coat dilution genes, resulting in an additive effect of the two loci. *CH* and *CR* alleles result in a very lightly colored horse similar to a creamello or perlino. In individuals with both a *CH* and *D* allele, the color is diluted but the *Dun* characteristics of a dorsal stripe and leg bands remain visible. As noted above, horses homozygous for the *prl* allele of *Cream Dilution* will appear very similar to heterozygotes for *CH*. Determining the genetic basis for the champagne color may require DNA testing. The effects of each possible genotype for the *Champagne Dilution* locus on the base coat colors is shown in Table 5.6.

Table 5.6. Genotypes and phenotypes for alleles of the *Champagne Dilution* gene (*CH*) with different base color phenotypes.

Base color phenotype (*E*, *A* loci)	*CH* genotype	Phenotypic effect
Chestnut	*chch*	Chestnut
	CHch	Gold champagne
	CHCH	Gold champagne
Bay	*chch*	Bay
	CHch	Amber champagne
	CHCH	Amber champagne
Black	*chch*	Black
	CHch	Classic champagne
	CHCH	Classic champagne

Molecular genetics and gene location

CH has been mapped to ECA14 (Cook *et al.*, 2008). Sequencing of the *SLC36A1* gene revealed a missense mutation that was completely associated with *CH*. *SLC36A1* is located at EquCab2 chr14:26,678,645-26,701,135. *CH* is due to a missense mutation resulting in the substitution of an amino acid in the second exon of *SLC36A1*.

Gene function

Notably, *CH* is the first phenotype attributed to the *SLC36A1* gene in any species. However, as it is similar in structure to the gene responsible for *C (SLC45A2)*, it is not surprising that the two genes have similar effects on pigmentation. The precise function of *SLC36A1* is not currently known. Evidence in rats suggests that it may be important for the maturation of melanosomes (Cook *et al.*, 2008). Further study of the *CH* phenotype will provide needed insight in to the function of *SLC36A*. Due to its dominant mode of inheritance, genetic testing is necessary to identify homozygotes with certainty. Several commercial labs now offer a test for the *CH* allele.

Breeds

CH is predominantly found in breeds developed in North America, such as the American Saddlebred, American Quarter Horse, Tennessee Walking horse, and Appaloosa.

References

Adalsteinsson, S. (1974) Inheritance of the palomino color in Icelandic horses. *Journal of Heredity* 65, 15–20.

Andersson, L.S., Juras, R., Ramsey, D.T., Eason-Butler, J., Ewart, S., Cothran, G. and Lindgren, G. (2008) Equine multiple congenital ocular anomalies maps to a 4.9 megabase interval on horse chromosome 6. *BMC Genetics* 9: 88, doi:10.1186/1471-2156-9-88.

Bowling, A.T. (1996) *Horse Genetics*. CAB International, Wallingford, UK.

Brunberg, E., Andersson, L., Cothran, G., Sandberg, K., Mikko, S. and Lindgren, G. (2006) A missense mutation in *PMEL17* is associated with the silver coat color in the horse. *BMC Genetics* 7: 46, doi:10.1186/1471-2156-7-46.

Castle, W.E. (1948) The ABC of color inheritance in horses. *Genetics* 33, 22–35.

Castle, W.E. and Smith, F.H. (1953) Silver dapple, a unique color variety among Shetland ponies. *Journal of Heredity,* 44, 139–145.

Clark, L.A., Wahl, J.M., Rees, C.A. and Murphy, K.E. (2006) Retrotransposon insertion in *SILV* is responsible for merle patterning of the domestic dog. *Proceedings of the National Academy of Sciences of the United States of America* 103, 1376–1381.

Cook, D., Brooks, S., Bellone, R. and Bailey, E. (2008) Missense mutation in exon 2 of *SLC36A1* responsible for champagne dilution in horses. *PLoS Genetics* 4(9): e1000195, doi:10.1371/journal.pgen.1000195.

Costin, G.E., Valencia, J.C., Vieira, W.D., Lamoreux, M.L. and Hearing, V.J. (2003) Tyrosinase processing and intracellular trafficking is disrupted in mouse primary melanocytes carrying the *underwhite* (*uw*) mutation. A model for oculocutaneous albinism (OCA) type 4. *Journal of Cellular Science*, 116, 3203–3212.

Gremmel, F. (1939) Coat color in horses. *Journal of Heredity*, 30, 437–445.

Gutiérrez-Gil, B., Wiener, P. and Williams, J.L. (2007) Genetic effects on coat colour in cattle: dilution of eumelanin and phaeomelanin pigments in an F2-Backcross Charolais × Holstein population. *BMC Genetics* 8: 56, doi: 10.1186/1471-2156-8-56.

Knottenbelt, D.C. and Pascoe, R.R. (1994) *Colour Atlas of Diseases and Disorders of the Horse*. Mosby-Year Book Europe Limited (now of Elsevier Science), London.

Locke, M.M., Ruth, L.S., Millon, L.V., Penedo, M.C., Murray, J.D. and Bowling, A.T. (2001) The *Cream Dilution* gene, responsible for the palomino and buckskin coat colours, maps to horse chromosome 21. *Animal Genetics* 32, 340–343.

Mariat, D., Taourit, S. and Guérin, G. (2003) A mutation in the *MATP* gene causes the cream coat colour in the horse. *Genetics Selection Evolution* 35, 119–133.

Schmutz, S.M. and Berryere, T.G. (2007) The genetics of cream coat color in dogs. *Journal of Heredity* 98, 544–548.

Sponenberg, D.P. (2009) *Equine Color Genetics*, 3rd edn. Wiley-Blackwell, Ames, Iowa.

Trommershausen-Smith, A., Suzuki, Y. and Stormont, C. (1976) Use of blood typing to confirm principles of coat-color genetics in horses. *Journal of Heredity* 67, 6–10.

Van Vleck, L.D. and Davitt, M. (1977) Confirmation of a gene for dominant dilution of horse colors. *Journal of Heredity* 68, 280–282.

Websites

UC Davis Veterinary Medicine, Veterinary Genetics Laboratory, University of California at Davis, California. Available at: http://www.vgl.ucdavis.edu/ (accessed 15 January 2013).

Services: Dun Zygosity Test. Available at: http://www.vgl.ucdavis.edu/services/dunhorse.php (accessed 15 January 2013).

Services: Pearl. Available at: http://www.vgl.ucdavis.edu/services/horse/pearl.php (accessed 10 December 2012).

6 Tobiano, White, Sabino, and Roan (*KIT*)

The set of genes for tobiano, sabino, white, and roan produces white hair against the basic color patterns of chestnut, bay, or black as determined by the *Extension* (*E*) locus modified by the *Agouti* (*A*) locus. While other genes can produce white hair patterns, as discussed in subsequent chapters, the four traits of tobiano, sabino, white, and roan are all products of the same gene, *KIT*. The genetics of each pattern were well known before the discovery of the common genetic element; consequently, they each were assigned unique genetic names: *Tobiano* (*TO*), *Sabino* (*SB1*), *Dominant White* (*W*), and *Roan* (*RN*). In many mammals, including the mouse and pig, dominantly inherited white spotting patterns are due to mutations of the *KIT* gene (Geissler *et al.*, 1988; Besmer *et al.*, 1993; Johansson Moller *et al.*, 1996). Although these diverse coat color patterns have a single molecular source, using separate genetic terminology for the four traits remains useful.

Tobiano

The inheritance of the tobiano pattern of white spotting is well known to be a dominant trait. A tobiano foal must have a tobiano parent. Fillies and colts inherit tobiano from either sire or dam, or both. The tobiano gene is absent in the predominant North American breeds of Quarter Horse, Thoroughbred, Standardbred and Arabian, but is found in a wide variety of other breeds, including Paint, Pinto, Dutch Warmblood, American Saddlebred, Tennessee Walking horse, Missouri Fox Trotter, Paso Fino, Icelandic, Shetland and Miniature.

The overall impression of a tobiano is that of a white horse on which large colored patches have been placed (Plate 9). The colored areas generally include the head, the chest, and the flanks. Pink skin underlies the white areas and there is black skin under the colored areas. The eyes are usually brown, but one or both may be blue or partially blue. The tail may be of two colors (white with black or red), a characteristic seldom seen in horses other than tobianos. The tobiano pattern is obvious at birth. Comparison of foal and adult photographs shows that the large pattern definition remains constant during the horse's lifetime, though the outlines of the markings may change in small details. To be registered as a tobiano Paint, a horse must meet the American Paint Horse Association (APHA) pedigree and requirements for white markings. The APHA describes the characteristic pattern features of tobiano as follows (see Website section for URL):

1. The dark color usually covers one or both flanks.
2. Generally, all four legs are white, at least below the hocks and knees.
3. Generally, the spots are regular and distinct as ovals or round patterns that extend down over the neck and chest, giving the appearance of a shield.

© E. Bailey and S.A. Brooks 2013. *Horse Genetics*, 2nd Edition (E. Bailey and S.A. Brooks)

4. Head markings are like those of a solid-colored horse – solid, or with a blaze, strip, star or snip.
5. A tobiano may be either predominantly dark or white.
6. The tail is often of two colors.

As with many patterns, the expression of the tobiano pattern can vary owing to the contribution of many unknown modifying genes. Individuals have been noted to carry the tobiano allele and possess remarkably minimal markings – generally white legs and some white in the mane or tail.

Combination with colors and other patterns

Tobiano can occur with any coat color (sorrel tobiano, bay tobiano, palomino tobiano, dun tobiano, black tobiano, and so on), and can also occur in a mixture with other spotting patterns. For instance, a combination of tobiano with overo ("tovero" or "medicine hat") results in a horse with more total white than either individual spotting gene could usually produce: an additive genetic effect. The interaction of *Tobiano* and *Overo* (see Chapter 8) genes can at its most extreme result in a white horse. Genes that produce leg and facial markings probably also interact with *Tobiano* to affect the extent of white (sabino, for example). A tobiano with a minimal white pattern may lack independently inherited genes for common white markings.

Tobiano can also occur in combination with roan (*RN*) and appaloosa (*LP*; see Chapter 9) spotting patterns. As neither the Paint nor the Appaloosa breed allows registration of tobiano/appaloosa pattern blends, the "pintaloosa" is perhaps the best known today as a color variant in American Miniature Horses and other breeds with no registration restrictions on pattern. Mule breeders have demonstrated that the best way to get fancy stockings on a mule is to use a tobiano mare. For mules with the *Tobiano* gene, the extent of body spots may be quite restricted compared with the expression of *Tobiano* in the horse parent, but the leg markings part of the pattern is consistently present.

Trait inheritance and gene symbol

The locus symbol for the *Tobiano* gene is *TO*, and we also use *TO* for the dominant allele of the pattern; the recessive allele, absence of tobiano spotting, uses *to*. The genotype for a horse with the tobiano pattern is either *TOTO* (homozygous) or *TOto* (heterozygous) (see Table 6.1). Homozygotes for *Tobiano* are usually indistinguishable from heterozygotes. However, homozygotes will always produce offspring with

Table 6.1. Phenotypes and genotypes for the *Tobiano* (*TO*) allele.

Phenotype	Genotype
Tobiano	*TOTO* or *Toto*
Non-tobiano	*toto*

tobiano spotting patterns and are highly valued by breeders. In the past, laboratories tested for genetic variants of two genes (*Albumin* and *Vitamin-D binding protein* (*GC*)) associated with the pattern, and used pedigree information to advise a breeder on the probability that their horse was homozygous for *Tobiano*. Today, a definitive genetic test is commercially available (Brooks *et al.*, 2007). Horses without the tobiano pattern gene are denoted as *toto*. This single dominant gene determines the appearance of the tobiano patterns; if a horse does not have the *TO* gene, it cannot pass the trait to its offspring, even if its parents had the tobiano pattern.

Tobianos often have a few, small, colored spots in white areas. Occasionally, tobiano horses show a dramatic proliferation of small, clustered spots, often with roan edges – "halos", or with roaning of the entire spot. Clustered colored spots that appear to be breaking through in otherwise large areas of body white have been called "ink spots" or "paw prints" (Plate 9). Horses that are homozygous for tobiano commonly have these spots, with a moderate extent of white area. Although dramatically evident at times, the association of ink spots with homozygosity does not appear to be absolute. Therefore, the best method for determining zygosity is by DNA testing. Only a horse with two copies of *Tobiano* (homozygous) will be true breeding for this pattern (see Table 6.1).

Molecular genetics and gene location

Tobiano results from a unique chromosome rearrangement on ECA3, rather than a base change within the *KIT* gene itself (Brooks *et al.*, 2007). The rearrangement resulted from a section of the ECA3 that "flipped" during a recombination event. This flip created a segment of the chromosome where the gene order is inverted relative to the order that is common in ECA3. The inversion spans nearly a third of the length of the chromosome, and likely causes spotting by separating the *KIT* gene from important regulatory sequences. Loss of control by these regulatory regions may disrupt *KIT* signaling used to control melanocyte migration across the embryo. As already mentioned, a genetic test is commercially available from several laboratories to detect the mutation causing the tobiano pattern.

The DNA test for *Tobiano* has been used to show a single and ancient origin of this pattern (Brooks *et al.*, 2007). All horses with the tobiano pattern carry precisely the same DNA inversion associated with *KIT*. Its broad distribution among breeds from around the world, especially those that do not select positively for spotting patterns, certainly suggests that the mutation must have been present early in the formation of these breeds. Recent work that tested DNA samples from ancient horses has revealed that *Tobiano* is in fact quite old, as it appears in a number of animals that lived some ~3500 years before the present (Ludwig *et al.*, 2009).

Breeds

The tobiano pattern occurs in breeds worldwide, although "pied" is the English language term, which is probably more often used outside the Americas. "Tobiano" appears to have been coined in South America, where it was traditionally used for distinctively spotted horses said to have descended from those brought by a Dutch emigrant named Tobias. In Britain, tobiano horses may be called "painted", "colored", "piebald" (white and black), "skewbald" (white and any single color but black) or "odd-colored" (white and two or more colors), without distinguishing any particular pattern. Besides the North American horse breeds with tobiano spotting listed at the beginning of this chapter, others worldwide include East Prussian Trakehners, and native ponies such as the Pottok from the Basque region of Spain, and the Mongolian pony of central Asia.

Dominant White

The "white" horse has been valued throughout history; it has a ceremonial status, and is frequently portrayed in art and mythology. However, horses popularly called white often are genetically *Gray* or homozygotes for the *Cream Dilution* gene (cremello). From a genetics standpoint, the genetic term "*White*" is strictly reserved for the dominant hereditary trait that produces horses with extensive white pigmentation from birth. But whereas the presence of the gene for *White* determines the presence of white color, the extent of white is highly variable. In practice, the extent of white coloration can vary from being complete, to being mostly white but with pigment in the tips of the ears, to being white with extensive patches of pigment along the back and tail. Consequently, *White* has sometimes been described as producing "sabino-style spotting" (Mau *et al.*, 2004; Sponenberg, 2009).

The effect of the *White* gene is distinguishable from white coloration caused by the *Gray* or *Cream Dilution* genes. Gray horses are born with pigmented hair that becomes white with age but the skin remains dark; white horses have white hair from birth, with pink skin. Cremello horses (*CRCR*) are more difficult to distinguish from the effect of the *White* gene because they have both the cream phenotype from birth, and the pink skin. Their eyes, though, are usually blue in contrast to the usually brown eyes found in white horses; sometimes subtle differences can also be seen in the hue of cream or white hair at transition zones around the head or on the legs (Plate 10).

The genetics of *White* are more complex than the genetics described for *Extension*, *Agouti*, the dilution genes, and *Tobiano*. While *Extension*, *Agouti*, *Cream*, *Silver*, *Champagne* and *Tobiano* are the result of single, specific mutations in the associated genes, *White* can be caused by many and independent mutations at different sites within the gene *KIT* (see Table 6.2). In general, mutations in *KIT* commonly result in white hair color, but the extent and distribution of the white hair is a product of the site and nature of the mutation.

Trait inheritance and gene symbol

The symbol *W* was used very early to represent *Dominant White* in horses (reviewed in Castle, 1948). As implied by the name, the gene causing white coloration is dominant, and therefore *W* is used for the allele responsible for white, and *w* is used for the recessive allele, the absence of white. All non-white horses have the genotype *ww*. Molecular studies of *KIT* and white pigmentation led to the definition of a series of alleles encoding white hair color, which were identified as *W1–W17* (Table 6.2;

Chapter 6

Table 6.2. *Dominant White* (*W*) alleles for the *KIT* gene, with their associated breeds, types of mutation and location on the *KIT* gene (adapted from Haase *et al.*, 2011).

Designation	Breed	Mutation type	Location on *KIT*
W1	Franches-Montagnes	Nonsense	Exon15
W2	Thoroughbred	Missense	Exon17
W3	Arabian	Nonsense	Exon4
W4	Camarillo White	Missense	Exon12
W5	Thoroughbred	Frameshift	Exon15
W6	Thoroughbred	Missense	Exon5
W7	Thoroughbred	Splice site	Intron2
W8	Icelandic	Splice site	Intron15
W9	Holstein	Missense	Exon12
W10	Quarter Horse	Frameshift	Exon7
W11	German Draft	Splice site	Intron20
W12	Thoroughbred	Deletion	Exon3
W13	Quarter Horse	Splice site	Intron17
W14	Thoroughbred	Deletion	Exon17
W15	Arabian	Missense	Exon10
W16	Oldenburger	Missense	Exon18
W17	Japanese Draft	Missense	Exon14
Other *KIT* variants			
SB1	Many	Splice variant	Intron16
TO	Many	Inversion	Intergenic

Haase *et al.*, 2007, 2009, 2011). However, breeders continue to use the simple terminology, *W* or *w*, because the different alleles are only distinguishable by DNA sequencing.

Homozygous lethal white

No living *WW* (homozygous) horse has been reported. Castle (1948) recounted that some breeders thought that *Dominant White* might be a homozygous embryonic lethal trait based on the absence of true-breeding, homozygous *White* horses. He suggested that homozygous white foals might be lost during pregnancy. Breeders might not even become aware that their white mare had become pregnant, depending on how early the mare lost the foal. Pulos and Hutt (1969) did an extensive breeding study in which they mated white horses to white horses, and observed the ratio of white to non-white offspring. According to Mendel, they should have seen a 3:1 ratio of white to non-white, but what they saw was a 2:1 ratio, suggesting that the homozygous offspring were lost as embryos. (*Dominant White* is described as an example of dominant lethal genes in Chapter 2.) The phenotypes and genotypes for *W* are shown in Table 6.3.

The DNA sequencing results (mutation types) shown in Table 6.2 offer a likely explanation for the homozygous lethality of *W*. Most mutations responsible for *W* are nonsense mutations, frameshift mutations or DNA deletions, all of which would destroy the possibility of producing a functional KIT protein. Horses with one *KIT* mutation might be viable, albeit with some white hair, because they would have at

Table 6.3. Phenotypes and genotypes for the *Dominant White (W)* series of alleles.

Phenotype	Genotype
White	*Ww*
Not white	*ww*
Embryonic lethal	*WW*

least one copy of functional protein. However, two dysfunctional copies could result in failure for an embryo to develop: an embryonic lethal. Conversely, some of these mutations may not destroy the function of *KIT*. Missense and splice site mutations, for example, have a more modest effect on gene function. They might leave intact the ability to make a functional KIT protein. Consequently, homozygotes for these white alleles might be viable, but we will not know this unless someone mates two white horses with those mutations.

Molecular genetics and gene location

The *KIT* gene, responsible for *W*, is found on ECA3, like the *Tobiano* gene. As shown in Table 6.2, the mutations responsible for the trait can occur throughout the gene. Most *W* alleles in the horse have been found spontaneously, i.e. they occur in just one founder individual, and the offspring of that individual. The result is a large number of unique alleles (17 to date, as shown in Table 6.2), all within the *KIT* gene (Haase *et al.*, 2007, 2009, 2011; Holl *et al.*, 2010). Each allele is independently responsible for a *W–* type phenotype, though there is significant variation in the spectrum of phenotypes within the *W* series. Many *W* alleles are specific to a breed, or to a family of horses, making prognostic DNA-based testing difficult without screening for all alleles, or making an educated guess as to which test is appropriate based on the target breed. While it is possible to test for *W* using a DNA test, the diversity of mutations makes this commercially impractical.

Breeds

The *W* alleles are rare in nearly all breeds of horses. The color has appeared among Thoroughbreds, Arabians, American Quarter Horses, Hanoverians, Icelandics, as well as several others, and is the founding characteristic of the Camarillo White horse (Haase *et al.*, 2011). The diversity of mutations found in the *KIT* gene suggests that it may be prone to mutation. In that case, the opportunity exists for novel alleles of the *W* series to appear in any breed of horse.

Health concerns

As with any depigmented horse, individuals with a *W* allele will be extra sensitive to sun exposure. Although abnormalities of other systems, such as the blood, and testes or ovaries, are frequently seen in mice with *W* alleles, no such issues have yet been observed in the horse (Haase *et al.*, 2010). The evidence for a homozygous lethal effect was discussed above and in Chapter 2.

Sabino (*Sabino1*)

The name sabino is given to a white spotting pattern characterized by tall irregular stockings and a blaze on the face. Many horses with this pattern also have a splotch of white on the belly or flank. Sabino horses often possess a mixture of white hairs interspersed with the base coat color in an effect that is similar to that of roan or gray. The borders of sabino white markings are often more jagged than that of a sock or blaze caused by a typical white marking gene. Sabino is often confused with other patterns, especially splashed white and overo. For example, in the registry for the Tennessee Walking horse there are many foundation horses recorded as "roan" that exhibit the characteristics of sabino patterning in photographs. Some of these horses were described anecdotally as "lit-up roan", giving credit to the flashy nature of their white socks.

The term *sabino* is Spanish, and in Spain it is used not only to denote this particular color of horse, but also to denote "from the ancient region of Sabine". The Sabine people inhabited the mountains just to the north of modern Rome, and the Sabines played an integral role in the early history of the Roman Empire. How this geographical region came to be associated with this particular color of horse is unknown.

The focus of this section is on one particular sabino pattern, found in a variety of horse breeds, many of which have ties to Spanish bloodlines. As described below, a genetic mutation was found in the gene *KIT* that appears to be responsible for the trait. All horses found to have this mutation have a sabino pattern, but the mutation is not present among Clydesdale horses, or among other horses exhibiting another sabino pattern, demonstrating that there are multiple genetic pathways to producing this phenotype.

Trait inheritance and gene symbol

As noted in the previous paragraph, the genetics of sabino are different in some breeds. Therefore, the gene for the trait described here was given the name *Sabino1* (*SB1*) as the first gene discovered for the sabino pattern. The gene is an incomplete dominant identified as *SB1*, with the absence of sabino identified as *sb1*. A single copy of the gene will produce the sabino pattern in a horse. These individuals possess the characteristic flashy socks and blaze. However, homozygotes (*SB1SB1*) are white or near white, while sometimes retaining pigmentation along the dorsal midline (Plate 11). The pattern is unique and distinct from similar phenotypes caused by the *W* series of alleles in that sabino alleles do not produce a homozygous lethal (*WW*) as *W* does. For this reason, sabino was given its own symbol, *SB1*, rather than using the *W* symbol, as suggested by precedence in mouse research (Besmer *et al.*, 1993). The phenotypes and genotypes associated with *SB1* are shown in Table 6.4.

Table 6.4. Genotypes and phenotypes for the *Sabino* (*SB1*) locus.

Phenotype	Genotype
White Sabino	*SB1SB1*
Sabino	*SB1sb1*
Not sabino	*Sb1sb1*

Molecular genetics and gene location

The allele responsible for the one type of sabino pattern (*SB1*) described here was discovered within the *KIT* gene on ECA3 (Brooks and Bailey, 2005). A single base change within the 16th intron alters the regulation of exon splicing, resulting in a proportion of the gene transcripts lacking the 17th exon (see bottom of Table 6.2). As splicing is not completely disrupted, and even homozygotes retain some transcripts with the normal sequence, health deficits have not been reported in *SB1* horses.

Breeds

SB1 is found in many breeds of horse, from Miniature horses and Shetland ponies, to mustangs and gaited breeds. This diverse breed distribution suggests that the mutation is ancient. Indeed, the very old roots of this sabino pattern were demonstrated by the work of Ludwig *et al.* (2009). By testing samples of DNA from ancient horses, these authors demonstrated that the *SB1* pattern was present in a horse that lived on the Siberian steppe approximately 5000 years ago.

Clydesdales have a characteristic sabino-type pattern, but *SB1* has not been found in this or in other draft breeds. Clearly, sabino in these breeds has a different genetic origin, possibly another mutation of *KIT*, or a consequence of a mutation at yet another locus.

Roan

The *Roan* gene produces a silvering effect by mixing white and colored hairs, generally more so on the body than the head and the lower legs (Plate 12). The roan effect does not progressively whiten with age as does gray, although often the summer coat appears lighter than the winter coat. Hair regrowth in areas of skin wounds may not show the white hair mixture, thus accentuating the appearance of scars (and brands) in the roan coat.

A wonderful array of names can be used for the color variations produced by the combinations of roan with the basic colors, but most breed registries limit the options. In some schemes, "blue roan" may be used as the color term for black, brown, or bay, with roan and "red roan" used for sorrel or chestnut with roan. Sometimes, bay with roan is called "strawberry roan". Other breeds simply register the horse as "roan", losing the record of the basic coat color. The presence of the roan allele is obvious by its silvering effect on coat color, and its inheritance follows a dominant pattern. However, a roan-type effect can be produced by other genes, which sometimes creates confusion in color designations for registration, and in assigning genotypes. For example, the gene responsible for leopard (*LP*, appaloosa) spotting may also produce a mottled roaning effect called varnished roan.

Trait inheritance and gene symbol

Roan is represented by the symbol "*RN*". The roan trait has a dominant mode of inheritance, and the dominant allele is represented by *RN*, with the recessive allele, absence of roan, represented as *rn*. No mutations have been identified for *RN*, even though the trait is associated with *KIT* (Marklund *et al.*, 1999). No commercial tests exist for detection of the *RN* gene either.

Homozygous lethal roan

Hintz and Van Vleck (1979) suggested that *RN* is a homozygous lethal gene after investigating the registry records for American-bred Belgian Draft horses. They discovered a deficit of roan patterned offspring of roan parents. Mendelian expectations predict a 3:1 ratio of roan to non-roan offspring; the ratio found by these authors was closer to 2:1, and consistent with embryonic loss of homozygotes for roan. But since then, there have been numerous anecdotal reports of homozygous, true-breeding roan stallions in the USA, Germany, and Japan; published reports of homozygous roan stallions include those of Geurts (1977), Bowling (2000), and Sponenberg (2009), particularly in the Quarter Horse. These conflicting accounts may eventually be explained should more than one *RN* allele be identified. Phenotypes and genotypes for the *RN* allele (showing both the possibility and non-occurrence of homozygous lethals) are shown in Table 6.5.

Roan variant: rabicano

Many horses have at least a few scattered white hairs, which could occasionally be confused with the actions of *RN*. Occasionally, a horse may have a heavy dose of roaning without having a roan parent to contribute an *RN* gene. For instance, in Arabian horses, among over 500,000 historical registrations in the Arabian Horse Registry of America (AHRA) Stud Book, 290 horses are designated as roan. Some of the roans are probably misidentified grays (*G*), particularly in early records. When

Table 6.5. Phenotypes and genotypes for the *Roan* (*RN*) alleles.

Phenotype	Genotype
Roan	*RNrn*
Not roan	*rnrn*
Lethal or Roan	*RNRN*

those with a *G* or an *RN* parent are excluded, there are still 73 horses with the roan designation. Based on the traditional definition of roan as a dominant gene, these data could be taken to suggest either a very high percentage of pedigree error among Arab roans, or a significant underreporting of the roan pattern. Parentage verification through genetic marker testing provides validation of the recent stud book records, and there is no compelling evidence to support the notion that parentage assignment would be grossly inaccurate among the older records. If underreporting of the roan color does occur, it is not likely to be deliberate as most breeders appreciate the traditional status of this pattern, and welcome its distinctiveness. Therefore, it seems likely that the action of another, recessive, allele may be creating a roan-like pattern. This "roaning" pattern is frequently called rabicano.

Compared with the classic roan gene, the rabicano trait is typically an uneven pattern, heavier on the flanks, and on the barrel, than on the forehand. Other prominent features include white flecking (irregularly shaped, white spots) on the flanks and belly, between the front and hind legs, and on the sides of the neck near where it joins the head. Particularly large flecked areas may be underlain with pink skin. The mixed coat may have a diffuse vertical white striping pattern reminiscent of brindling in dogs or cattle. Often the hair on the top of the tail is white, perhaps with several rows of prominent stripes across the top of the dock. The rabicano trait is not confined to Arabians, but is found in many breeds, including Thoroughbred horses and Quarter Horses. The inheritance of rabicano has not been defined.

Molecular genetics and gene location

The gene coding for *RN* appears to be on ECA3, near or within the *KIT* gene. Sequencing *KIT* exons did not reveal the mutation responsible for *RN*, but the studies did demonstrate that *RN* might be a mutation within or nearby the *KIT* gene (Marklund *et al.*, 1999). Per se, this result also suggests that *RN* is part of the genetic series including *Tobiano*, *White*, and *Sabino*, and may be listed in Table 6.2. As already noted, no commercial tests exist for detection of the *RN* gene.

Breeds

The *RN* allele is found in such diverse breeds as the Quarter Horse, Peruvian Paso, Paso Fino, Welsh pony, Miniature, and Belgian. The term "roan" is used for the assigned color in stud book and racetrack descriptions of some Thoroughbreds with bay and grey, as a way to distinguish them from those with chestnut and grey, thus contributing to confusion about the definition of "roan". Roan is recognized as a color in the Arabian stud book, but in this breed an extensive interspersed white hair pattern may be due to another gene or genes.

We may discover that *RN* is not the result of a single mutation in a single gene, but occurs as a consequence of different mutations in different breeds, like the *W* allele series. This would be consistent with the nature of *KIT* mutations, and would explain the subtle phenotypic differences that are found, such as rabicano. Furthermore, it might explain why some *RN* alleles are homozygous lethal and others may be viable as homozygotes: mutations such as deletions would destroy KIT protein production, while missense mutations might produce the roan phenotype and also allow the production of KIT protein. The former case would result in an embryonic lethal, whereas the latter case could result in a viable pregnancy.

Summary

KIT mutations play a key role in producing white spotting patterns in horses. However, not all white spotting patterns in horses are products of the *KIT* locus. The next few chapters describe the genetics of the traits gray, overo, splashed white and leopard, all of which are encoded by genes elsewhere in the genome. Nevertheless, the diversity of mutations and phenotypes that occur associated with *KIT* are remarkable. The association of *KIT* with white spotting is not confined to horses, of course, and we draw on a remarkable body of knowledge about the genetics of *KIT* and melanogenesis in other species, and especially from studies in mice (Geissler *et al.*, 1988; Besmer *et al.*, 1993; Johansson Moller *et al.*, 1996). As noted above, we still have not identified the mutations responsible for sabino in draft horses, nor the mutations for roan patterns. The work of Marklund *et al.* (1999) indicated that at least one of the *RN* mutations is associated with *KIT*, but it remains possible that mutations in other genes can create the roan phenotype – or the sabino phenotype of draft horses.

References

Besmer, P., Manova, K., Duttlinger, R., Huang, E.J., Packer, A., Gyssler, C. and Bachvarova, R.F. (1993) The kit-ligand (steel factor) and its receptor c-kit/W: pleiotropic roles in gametogenesis and melanogenesis. *Development* (Supplement 1993), 125–137.

Bowling, A.T. (2000) Genetics of colour variation. In: Bowling, A.T. and Ruvinsky, A. (eds) *The Genetics of the Horse.* CAB International, Wallingford, UK, pp. 53–70.

Brooks, S.A. and Bailey, E. (2005) Exon skipping in the *KIT* gene causes a Sabino spotting pattern in horses. *Mammalian Genome* 16, 893–902.

Brooks, S.A., Lear, T.L., Adelson, D.L. and Bailey, E. (2007) A chromosome inversion near the *KIT* gene and the Tobiano spotting pattern in horses. *Cytogenetic and Genome Research* 119, 225–230.

Castle, W.E. (1948) The ABC of color inheritance in the horse. *Genetics* 33, 22–35.

Geissler, E.N., Ryan, M.A. and Housman, D.E. (1988) The dominant-white spotting (*W*) locus of the mouse encodes the c-*kit* proto-oncogene. *Cell* 55, 185–192.

Guerts, R. (1977) *Hair Colour in the Horse.* J.A. Allen, London.

Haase, B., Brooks, S.A., Schlumbaum, A., Azor, P.J., Bailey, E., Alaeddine, F., Mevissen, M., Burger, D., Poncet, P.-A., Rieder, S. and Leeb, T. (2007) Allelic heterogeneity at the equine *KIT* locus in dominant white (*W*) horses. *PLoS Genetics* 3(11): e195, doi:10.1371/journal.pgen.0030195.

Haase, B., Brooks, S.A., Tozaki, T., Burger, D., Poncet, P.-A., Rieder, S., Hasegawa, T., Penedo, C. and Leeb, T. (2009) Seven novel *KIT* mutations in horses with white coat colour phenotypes. *Animal Genetics* 40, 623–629.

Haase, B., Obexer-Ruff, G., Dolf, G., Rieder, S., Burger, D., Poncet, P.-A., Gerber, V., Howard, J. and Leeb, T. (2010) Haematological parameters are normal in dominant white Franches-Montagnes horses carrying a *KIT* mutation. *Veterinary Journal* 184, 315–317.

Haase, B., Rieder, S., Tozaki, T., Hasegawa, T., Penedo, M.C., Jude, R. and Leeb, T. (2011) Five novel *KIT* mutations in horses with white coat colour phenotypes. *Animal Genetics* 42, 337–339.

Hintz, R.L. and Van Vleck, L.D. (1979) Lethal dominant roam in horses. *Journal of Heredity* 70, 145–146.

Holl, H., Brooks, S. and Bailey, E. (2010) *De novo* mutation of *KIT* discovered as a result of a non-hereditary white coat color pattern. *Animal Genetics* 41, 196–198.

Johansson Moller, M., Chaudhary, R., Hellmen, E., Hoyheim, B., Chowdhary, B. and Andersson, L. (1996) Pigs with the dominant white coat color phenotype carry a duplication of the *KIT* gene encoding the mast/stem cell growth factor receptor. *Mammalian Genome* 7, 822–830.

Ludwig, A., Pruvost, M., Reissmann, M., Benecke, N., Brockmann, G.A., Castanos, P., Cieslak, M., Lippold, S., Llorente, L., Malaspinas, A.S., Slatkin, M. and Hofreiter, M. (2009) Coat color variation at the beginning of horse domestication. *Science* 324, 485.

Marklund, S., Moller, M., Sandberg, K. and Andersson, L. (1999) Close association between sequence polymorphism in the *KIT* gene and the roan coat color in horses. *Mammalian Genome* 10, 283–288.

Mau, C., Pondet, P.-A., Bucher, B., Stranzinger, G. and Rieder, S. (2004) Genetic mapping of *Dominant White* (*W*), a homozygous lethal condition in the horse (*Equus caballus*). *Journal of Animal Breeding Genetics* 1221, 374–383.

Pulos, W.L. and Hutt, F.B. (1969) Lethal dominant white in horses. *Journal of Heredity* 60, 59–63.

Sponenberg, D.P. (2009) *Equine Color Genetics*, 3rd edn. Wiley-Blackwell, Ames, Iowa.

Website

American Paint Horse Association (APHA), Fort Worth, Texas. The Breed: Tobiano. Available at: http://www.apha.com/breed/tobiano (accessed 15 January 2013).

7 Gray

Everyone is familiar with the progressive changes of human hair color in which the hair color of youth is replaced with gray or white. Horses show a similar phenomenon of hair silvering, although it occurs at a proportionately much younger age than in people. A young horse that has the progressive graying allele can be born any color. In the popular literature, the birth color of grays is often said to be black, but that is not true for all breeds. The birth color of a gray horse is a function of the alleles of the other coat color genes of that individual, particularly *Agouti* and *Extension*. For example, most gray Arabians are born bay or chestnut, not black.

The Gray Trait

Soon after birth a foal going gray will begin to show intermixed white hairs that proportionally increase in number with age. The rate at which this change will occur is dependent on a number of factors, primarily the base coat color. Chestnut (*ee*) base color horses will acquire white hairs at a much faster rate than darker base color horses (Rosengren Pielberg *et al.*, 2008). Other unknown heritable factors also impact the rate of pigmentation loss and are unique to some breeds. For example, the Arabian horse stud book records made on the basis of foal colors at about 6 months of age will often accurately reflect the gray color of the mature horse. In contrast, this same determination is not always possible at 6 months of age in other breeds such as the Thoroughbred. At intermediate stages, many gray horses show a dappling pattern of light gray hair splotches surrounded by dark gray rings. The knees, hocks and fetlocks may be obviously dark gray, a character usually retained for longer than dappling. At maturity, the hair coat will be a clear gray (it appears as a "pure" white horse with dark skin; see Plate 13) or gray with colored speckling ("flea-bitten" or "mosquito-bitten"). Some chestnuts going gray proceed through a stage known as "rose gray". "Dun-like" markings, often faint in other colors, may be quite prominent in intermediately gray foals.

Care must be taken during the registration process to distinguish those white markings on a gray horse that have underlying pink skin from those that do not. Particularly around the face, white markings may not be accompanied by pink skin, and in a mature gray horse such markings will no longer be visible. White spotting patters such as tobiano, overo and appaloosa may not be readily visible as a coat pattern in a mature gray horse, but can be seen as pink skin patterns, particularly when the hair is wet.

Trait inheritance and gene symbol

The locus symbol for the *Gray* gene is *G*, and the dominant allele for *Gray* is designated *G*, while the recessive allele for non-gray is *g*. A gray horse will be either *GG* or *Gg* (Table 7.1). It is not possible to tell by looking at the horse whether it is homozygous for *G*. A horse without the *Gray* gene is symbolized as *gg*. *Gray* interacts epistatically with all other coat color genes except white, obscuring their actions so that it is difficult or impossible to determine by looking at a gray horse what other coat color genes it possesses.

The earliest indications of the presence of the *G* allele can be seen by careful study of the head of a young foal, particularly around the eyes. Later, the horse will have a mixture of white and dark hairs throughout the body, a stage that can easily be confused with roan. Foals with the *G* allele are frequently born with a much darker base color than their not-gray counterparts. For example, the foal coat of a chestnut is often a light fawn color, which is particularly evident on the legs, but will later shed to produce the darker adult shade. Newborn chestnut foals carrying a *Gray* allele appear to possess the dark chestnut color of an adult but will later lose this hue during the change to gray. The foal coat darkening effect of *G–* appears to affect all base colors. Bay foals also typically have fawn-colored hair on their legs, which sheds to produce black. In bay foals that are going to be gray, the legs are black at birth. Black horses with *G* are born a shiny black, rather than the more typical mouse-gray foal color of blacks.

As gray color is produced by the action of a dominant gene, at least one parent of a gray horse must be gray. If a gray horse does not have a gray parent, then the purported parentage is likely to be incorrect (Trommershausen-Smith *et al.*, 1976). A foal with two gray parents has at least a 25% chance to be homozygous for gray. Homozygous grays, as with other dominant alleles, should only have gray offspring. When an apparent exception occurs in the stud book, usually it is found that the horse is gray but the owner did not recognize the color when filling out registration forms and failed to notify the stud book in time to change the published color.

The color nomenclature for gray can be confusing. In the case of the Thoroughbred stud book, grays born chestnut are customarily registered as "roan", while grays born dark bay, brown or black are registered as "gray". Bays with *G–* may be called either "roan" or "gray", depending on how conspicuous is the red hair component. (The classic roan gene, per se, is not found in Thoroughbreds.)

The incidence of speckling ("flea-bites") varies greatly among individuals and breeds possessing the gray allele. No genetic analysis for independent inheritance for the speckling trait in grays has been reported. However, the gray genotype does seem to have a considerable impact on the appearance of speckles. Horses that are *GG* homozygous usually do not possess speckles once the graying process is complete.

Table 7.1. Genotypes and phenotypes for the *Gray* gene.

Phenotype	Genotype
Gray	*Gg, GG*
Not gray	*gg*

Most speckled horses are *Gg* heterozygous. Alleles that are common only to certain breeds may also play a part as breeds in which gray is rare (so most horses are heterozygous), and these usually do not possess speckles. Likewise, a non-flecked heterozygous gray bred to a *gg* (not-gray) may have flecked gray offspring. This situation suggests that speckling is a trait separate from gray, yet interacts with the gray allele.

Gray horses are also susceptible to a progressive loss of pigmentation in the skin known as vitiligo. This depigmentation occurs around the eyes, mouth, and anus, and although it is frequently considered unattractive, it is not a health risk. This can be a frustration to owners because in some horses the condition disappears and in others it persists. As with melanomas, vitiligo depigmentation is also occasionally seen with other colors, but it is more often associated with gray. Vitiligo may be a hereditary trait genetically independent of *Gray*, but which may interact (epistatically) with the *Gray* gene.

Molecular genetics and gene location

The gene for *Gray* was mapped to ECA25 independently by three research groups (Henner *et al.*, 2002; Locke *et al.*, 2002; Swinburne *et al.*, 2002). The duplication of 4200 bp of sequence within an intron of the *STX17* gene was subsequently shown to cause *G* (Rosengren Pielberg *et al.*, 2008). Consequently, there is a commercially available DNA test for *Gray*.

Gene function

STX17 is a member of the syntaxin protein family, a group with important functions in the targeting of vesicles and membrane trafficking. Although the expression of both *STX17* and a neighboring gene, *NR4A3*, is increased by presence of the *G* duplication, neither gene offers a simple explanation for how this change led to the gray phenotype (Rosengren Pielberg *et al.*, 2008). Subsequent experiments examining the sequence of the duplication revealed that it possessed regulatory sequences specific to melanocytes and acting on the neighboring *NR4A3* gene (Sundström *et al.*, 2012). Additional research is needed, but as *NR4A3* is important for regulating the cell cycle, it now seems likely that upregulation due to the *G* duplication could cause exhaustion of the melanocyte population in the hair follicle (leading to pigment loss with age), and overgrowth of some melanocyte populations in the skin (resulting in tumors).

All gray horses have this particular mutation. While we have the DNA sequence, we still do not know why horses become gray at different ages, or exhibit the diversity of secondary characteristics described above. These other characteristics may be the result of yet other genes acting in concert with *Gray*.

Breeds

Gray occurs in breeds throughout the world, including ponies, riding horses and draft horses. It is the predominant, but not exclusive, color in a few breeds (e.g. Andalusian,

Kladruber, and Lipizzaner). This widespread breed distribution suggests a fairly ancient origin for the gray color.

Health concerns

Gray horses are susceptible to a particular type of tumor that, although it originates with pigment-producing melanocyte cells, is not caused by exposure to the sun as are most human melanomas. In this case, the duplication responsible for the gray color may also alter the regulation of the cell cycle in dermal pigment cells, resulting in overgrowth and the development of tumors. Equine melanomas in non-gray horses are very rare. The tumors are most commonly seen around the tail or the head, but are occasionally found internally in any organ system. Gray horse melanomas are benign, but may be disfiguring and can lead to loss of use of the associated body part if the tumor causes discomfort or becomes ulcerated (Seltenhammer *et al.*, 2003). Internal tumors can be life-threatening if they interfere with vital organ function. Gray horses that also possess the *Agouti* (aka *ASIP*) genotype *aa* (black) are more likely to develop melanoma than those with *Aa* or *AA* (Rosengren Pielberg *et al.*, 2008). The *ASIP* genotype does not alter the rate of melanoma development in gray horses with the chestnut (*ee*) genotype, owing to the loss of *MC1R* function (and black pigmentation) conferred by the *e* (*Extension*) allele.

References

Henner, J., Poncet, P.-A., Guérin, G., Hagger, C., Stranzinger, G. and Rieder, S. (2002) Genetic mapping of the (*G*)-locus, responsible for the coat color phenotype "progressive greying with age" in horses (*Equus caballus*). *Mammalian Genome* 13, 535–537.

Locke, M.M., Penedo, M.C.T., Bricker, S.J., Millon, L.V. and Murray, J.D. (2002) Linkage of the grey coat color locus to microsatellites on horse chromosome 25. *Animal Genetics* 33, 329–337.

Rosengren Pielberg, G. *et al.* (2008) A *cis*-acting regulatory mutation causes premature hair graying and susceptibility to melanoma in the horse. *Nature Genetics* 40, 1004–1009.

Seltenhammer, M.H., Simhofer, H., Scherzer, S., Zechner, R., Curik, I., Solkner, J., Brandt, S.M., Jansen, B., Pehamberger, H. and Eisenmenger, E. (2003) Equine melanoma in a population of 296 grey Lipizzaner horses. *Equine Veterinary Journal* 35, 153–157.

Sundström, E., Komisarczuk, A.Z., Jiang, L., Golovko, A., Navratilova, P., Rinkwitz, S., Becker, T.S. and Andersson, L. (2012) Identification of a melanocyte-specific, microphthalmia-associated transcription factor-dependent regulatory element in the intronic duplication causing hair greying and melanoma in horses. *Pigment Cell and Melanoma Research* 25, 28–36.

Swinburne, J.E., Hopkins, A. and Binns, M.M. (2002) Assignment of the horse gray coat color gene to ECA25 using whole genome scanning. *Animal Genetics* 33, 338–342.

Trommershausen-Smith, A., Suzuki, Y. and Stormont, C. (1976) Use of blood typing to confirm principles of coat-color genetics in horses. *Journal of Heredity* 67, 6–10.

8 Frame Overo and Splashed White

The nomenclature for white spotting in horses varies from region to region, influenced by the language and patterns in local horse breeds. Overo ("bird's egg pattern") is the term used in South America for a pattern that is often called sabino in North America. In the British Isles, terms are less discriminating and "painted", "piebald", "coloured", and "skewbald" can include tobiano patterns as well as overo-type patterns. Thus, there is significant variation in the terms used to describe these patterns, which often have no relationship to the underlying genetic mechanisms. Indeed, breeders generally appreciate that the patterns are hereditary but complex. Only when specific patterns are identified accurately in families or in breeds can the genetic basis be investigated. In this chapter, the genetic bases are described for two well-known white spotting patterns: frame overo and splashed white.

Frame Overo

The overall impression of a frame overo is that of a colored horse with white patches (Plate 14). Pink skin underlies the areas of white. The eyes are usually brown, but one or both may be blue or partially blue. The frame overo pattern is obvious at birth and does not change significantly over the lifetime of the horse. The American Paint Horse Association (APHA) is one of the breed registries that is based on spotting patterns. To be registered as an "overo" Paint, a horse must meet APHA pedigree and requirements for white markings. The APHA describes the characteristic "overo" pattern features as follows:

- The white usually will not cross the back of the horse between its withers and its tail.
- Generally, at least one and often all four legs will be of the dark color.
- Generally, the white is irregular, rather scattered or splashy. It is often referred to as calico.
- Head markings are predominantly white; often bald, apron or bonnet faced.
- An overo horse may be either predominantly dark or white. (The darker color is more common.)
- The tail is usually one color.

The above characteristics also encompass a broad variety of patterns. Among APHA's Paint horses, the most prominent and distinctive overo pattern is that of frame overo, in which the dark color typically occurs along the topline, chest, legs, and tail, with white occurring in a horizontal motif on the body, accompanied by substantial white face markings.

Overo can occur with any coat color (sorrel overo, bay overo, palomino overo, dun overo, black overo, and so on), and with other patterns. "Tovero" is used to describe the tobiano and overo composite; however, at the same time, tovero is often used to include composites of tobiano with a wide range of white patterns, including sabino, frame overo, and splashed white. A horse with genes for both patterns usually has more white area than colored area. Overo can also occur in combination with various appaloosa spotting patterns, but neither the Paint nor Appaloosa breed allows the registration of overo/appaloosa spotting blends.

Some people see tobianos as white horses with dark patches, and overos with the opposite scheme. In minimally marked tobianos, the white body markings generally appear as vertical stripes, but in overos the white patches more often show a horizontal spreading. Exceptions to these generalizations occur often, particularly when multiple spotting genes occur in one horse.

Notably, individuals carrying a frame overo allele do not always express the spotting pattern. This phenomenon is known as reduced penetrance; a special case in which the phenotype is not always expressed even when the allele is present. The degree of phenotypic penetrance may depend on the action of epistatic and modifying loci. In the case of the frame overo, incomplete penetrance can lead to the misclassification of individuals as solid or breeding stock and, occasionally, the appearance of an overo lethal white syndrome-affected foal from a "solid" colored parent (Lightbody, 2002).

Trait inheritance and gene symbol

The locus symbol for the *Frame Overo* gene is "*O*", but different texts have also used "*Ov*", "*OV*", "*FR*" and "*FrO*". The phenotypes and genotypes associated with the *Frame Overo* are shown in Table 8.1. The symbol "*O*" is used to designate the dominant allele responsible for the frame overo pattern, and the absence of the allele is designated as "*o*". However the gene action is more accurately described as incomplete dominance because there is a clear difference between homozygotes and heterozygotes for O. Individuals with one copy of *O* display the distinctive frame overo pattern described above. Individuals with two copies of *O* exhibit the lethal condition of overo lethal white syndrome (OLWS). As described below, foals homozygous for O are viable through pregnancy but at birth appear almost completely white and exhibit multiple developmental abnormalities. Such foals die shortly after birth. (A description of this tragic disease can be found below.)

Confusion resulting from the generic use of the term "overo" may lead to unnecessary euthanasia of white foals resulting from parents with overo-type or overo-like patterns. *Sabino1* (see Chapter 6), for example, is sometimes referred to as overo-type

Table 8.1. Genotypes and phenotypes for the *O* (*Frame Overo*) allele.

Phenotype	Genotype
Non-overo	*oo*
Frame overo	*Oo*
Overo lethal white syndrome (OLWS)	*OO*

pattern, but in stark contrast, homozygotes for *SB1* are healthy white foals. *O* is a homozygous lethal gene while homozygotes for *SB1* and *CR* (cremello) have similar phenotypes but are viable and healthy.

Molecular genetics and gene location

Several research groups have mapped the *Frame Overo* gene to ECA17 and identified a missense mutation in the *EDNRB* gene that is responsible for both the frame overo pattern and OLWS (Metallinos *et al.*, 1998; Santschi *et al.*, 1998; Yang *et al.*, 1998). The dinucleotide change resulting from the *O* mutation switches an amino acid from isoleucine to lysine in the genetic code of the endothelin receptor type B gene (*EDNRB*), and disrupts its function. *EDNRB* is located at chr17:50,604,167-50,625,930 in the EquCab2 genome assembly. As frame overo patterns can appear similar to other inherited patterns, testing for the mutation in *EDNRB* is the best way to be confident that the color pattern seen actually is frame overo. The *O* allele is easily detected, and a suitable genetic test is widely available. This test is applicable for unambiguously identifying carriers of the frame overo allele, as well as diagnosing suspected cases of OLWS.

Gene function

As noted above, the switch from isoleucine to lysine caused by the dinucleotide change in *O* disrupts the function of the *EDNRB* gene, and the resulting changed endothelin receptor type B protein is unable to fulfill its usual role. Under normal conditions, this function is important in the signaling for several types of neural crest-derived cells, including melanocytes and a specialized subset of nerve cells in the digestive tract (intestinal ganglia). Mammalian pigment cells (melanocytes) originate in the neural crest region of the early embryo and migrate during later developmental stages to populate selected areas throughout the body. Signaling through the *EDNRB* system is just one of many biological pathways that contribute to this migration. The loss of some *EDNRB* signaling in *Oo* animals results in the failure of melanocytes to fully migrate and reach certain areas of the body, thereby creating the visible overo pattern. Melanocytes are entirely lacking in the skin of foals affected with OLWS (Lightbody, 2002). Although intestinal ganglia precursor cells also rely on *EDNRB* signaling to migrate, in *Oo* horses they seem to complete their migration sufficiently to provide normal gut function. However, in *OO* horses, the loss of *EDNRB* signaling completely prevents migration, leading to a loss of ganglion cells and gut function.

Breeds

The frame overo pattern seems to occur in breeds worldwide, although it is not as common as the sabino patterns. It is frequently observed in the American Paint Horse, Pinto, American Mustang and American Miniature Horse. The *O* allele also exists in the Thoroughbred breed, although it is very rare.

Health concerns

Frame overos with blue eyes and extensive white areas on the face can be sensitive to the sun and owners report that these horses actively seek protective shade in summer (photophobia). Pink-skinned areas of the face, as with any pattern of depigmentation, are susceptible to sunburn and may require extra protection when they are turned out.

Occasional blue-eyed white foals (or nearly white foals with a few colored spots about the muzzle, ears, or tail) from overo-type parents have been noted for decades (Smith, 1977; Hultgren, 1982; Vonderfecht *et al.*, 1983). Nearly all show symptoms of intestinal discomfort within a few hours of birth, similar to the signs in a foal with retained meconium. Neither medication nor surgery is successful in overcoming the blockage. These foals cannot pass food through the digestive tract, either because of the lack of intestinal ganglia that control the peristaltic muscle actions of the gut or, more rarely, because of missing sections of the intestinal tract (ileocolonic aganglionosis). The disease is termed overo lethal white syndrome (OLWS). Nearly all affected foals are the products of the mating of phenotypically frame overo parents, but a rare few exceptions are reported, especially in cases of incomplete penetrance. The association of a neurological defect with a conspicuous and unusual pigment pattern is encountered in several other species. This results from the shared signaling pathways of migratory cells that originate from the same neural crest area during embryological development, in this case nerve cells (ganglia) and pigment cells (melanocytes).

Based on our knowledge of the inheritance of O, the likelihood of producing a frame overo or OLWS foal is simple to predict. Crossing an *oo*, non-overo, horse with an *Oo*, frame overo, mate will result in 50% of offspring bearing the *Oo* genotype (and the frame overo pattern) and 50% bearing *oo* (non-overo). In the case of two *Oo* parents, the result can be illustrated by a Punnett square (Table 8.2). The three genotypic classes fit a model of O as a dominant gene, with lethal effects in the homozygous condition. This model predicts that 25% of foals will be affected by OLWS. Notably, in the case of frame overo it does not pay off to cross "like to like". In each case a maximum of 50% of foals will carry the desirable frame overo pattern, but in mating two frame overo parents one out of four offspring will be lost to OLWS.

Table 8.2. Predicted genotypes for a cross of two heterozygous frame overo (*Oo*) horses.

Genetic contribution from *Oo* mare	Offspring characteristic	Genetic contribution from *Oo* stallion	
		O	*o*
O	Offspring genotype	OO	Oo
	Offspring phenotype	OLWS[a]	Frame overo
	Proportion of offspring	25%	25%
o	Offspring genotype	Oo	oo
	Offspring phenotype	Frame overo	Non-overo
	Proportion of offspring	25%	25%

[a]OLWS, overo lethal white syndrome.

Researchers seeking to identify the gene responsible for OLWS began with a similar condition in humans: Hirschsprung disease (aganglionic megacolon). This condition is due to many different mutations in the *EDNRB* gene. Hirschsprung disease differs from the horse problem in that it does not frequently involve a pigment disorder and can often be surgically corrected (Puffenberger *et al.*, 1994). The *spotted lethal* rat and *piebald* mouse also provide excellent models for frame overo, as both are characterized by spotting patterns and megacolon resulting from *EDNRB* mutations.

A lethal intestinal defect similar to that of OLWS has been reported in Clydesdale foals (Murray *et al.*, 1988; Dyke *et al.*, 1990). The foals, aged 4–9 months, had a history of lethargy and abdominal distention. The intestinal defect was characterized as megacolon and microscopic examination of the affected gut showed an absence of ganglia. This Clydesdale problem is different from OLWS in that the foals were not white and were not neonates. However, a sabino pattern is prominent in Clydesdales, so a connection of the intestinal defect to their spotting pattern is a distinct possibility.

Splashed White

"Splashed white" is a spotting phenotype in which the mode of appearance is of a horse that has been splashed with white paint from underneath (Plate 15). The pattern is characterized by white patches across the extremities, usually including all four lower limbs, the belly, and across the face (Klemola, 1933; Sponenberg, 2009). Face markings often include a broad blaze or bonnet, and blue or part-colored eyes. In contrast to the sabino and dominant white alleles of the *KIT* locus, these white markings are often contained within crisp borders, and leave the remaining areas pigmented without speckling or roaning. The quantity of depigmentation is variable in the splashed white pattern. Some splashed white individuals are very minimally marked, and the marks can be easily confused with common socks/blaze markings. A hereditary aspect to this condition has been widely accepted.

Trait Inheritance and gene symbol

The symbols *SW* and *Spl* have been used to represent a putative gene causing splashed white patterns. However, studies in a Quarter Horse family followed by investigations of other horses with splashed white led to discovery of two different genes responsible for some of the splashed white phenotypes (Hauswirth *et al.*, 2012). Consequently, genetic designations for the trait need to be made in association with molecular genetic tests.

One of the genes implicated for splashed white was *MITF*, whose product is the microphthalmia-associated transcription factor protein (MITF) (Hauswirth *et al.*, 2012). The *MITF* allele that does not cause spotting can be designated *MITF+*. The mutations causing splashed white phenotypes are dominant to the wild type MITF allele. Three mutations of *MITF* were found to be associated with splashed white: *MITF-prom1* (spotted, splashed white), *MITF-C280Sfs*20* (spotted, splashed white), and *MITF-N310S* (a spotting pattern called macchiato). The allele designations refer to the molecular changes and, respectively, represent a mutation in promoter 1 (insertion), a frameshift (deletion), and a missense mutation altering an amino acid in the MITF protein. For the purposes of commercial testing *MITF-prom1* and *MITF-C280Sfs*20* are referred to as *SW1* and *SW3*. As the Macchiato pattern was unique and occurred as a result of a spontaneous mutation in a single, sterile stallion, it is unlikely to be observed in other horses, and an abbreviated name has not been given to this allele (*Macchiato*). The alleles referred to as *SW3* and *Macchiato* are both very rare, and homozygotes have not been observed. The genotypes and phenotypes associated with *MITF* are shown in Table 8.3.

A second locus found to cause the splashed white phenotype was for the gene *PAX3*, whose product is the Paired Box 3 Transcription Factor (Hauswirth *et al.*, 2012). The normal allele, *PAX+*, does not cause spotting and is recessive to the dominant allele that causes the splashed white pattern, *PAX3-C70Y*. For the purposes of commercial testing, Hauswirth *et al.* (2012) referred to this allele as *SW2*. The genotypes and phenotypes for *PAX3* are shown in Table 8.4.

Healthy, *SW1* homozygous horses have been observed, as well as compound heterozygotes in combination with the *SW2* allele. These individuals have more extensive white areas than heterozygotes, exemplifying an additive mode of inheritance. The *SW3* allele is very rare, if not unique, and its interaction with other alleles is unknown. Hauswirth *et al.* (2012) observed homozygotes for *SW1* that were quite healthy but speculated that homozygotes for *SW2* and *SW3* would be embryonic lethal combinations based on the effect of similar mutations in mice.

Molecular genetics and gene location

MITF is located at ECA16:20,089,347-20,170,130 in the EquCab2 genome assembly, while *PAX3* is at ECA6:11,340,602-11,431,275. The genes were discovered following

Table 8.3. Genotypes and phenotypes for the splashed white (*SW*) *MITF* locus.

Phenotype	Genotype
No splash white	*MITF+/MITF+*
Splashed white (SW1)	*MITF-prom1/MITF+*
Splashed white (SW3)	*MITF-C280Sfs*20/MITF+*
Splashed white (Macchiato)	*MITF-N310S/MITF+*
Extensive splashed white	*MITF-prom1/MITF-prom1*
Not observed (lethal?)	*MITF-C280Sfs*20/MITF-C280Sfs*20*
Not observed	*MITF-N310S/MITF-N310S*

Table 8.4. Genotypes and phenotypes for the splashed white (*SW2*) *PAX3* locus.

Phenotype	Genotype
No splashed white	*PAX3+/PAX3+*
Splashed white (SW2)	*PAX3-C70Y/PAX3+*
Not observed (lethal?)	*PAX3-C70Y/PAX3-C70Y*

a genome-widescan in a Quarter Horse family segregating for splashed white, which implicated genes in these regions of ECA6 and ECA16. In these two regions, *MITF* and *PAX3* were obvious candidate genes because they caused similar phenotypes in mice and people. Sequencing horses with splashed white in different breeds led to discoveries of the different mutations that are involved.

Gene function

The *MITF* gene produces the microphthalmia-associated transcription factor, which is a protein signal responsible for triggering the transcription of genomic DNA into RNA in a number of genes, usually in response to a developmental or environmental trigger. One of the many targets of *MITF* is *KIT* (see Chapter 6), which important for melanocyte development. Therefore, it seems likely that, as in other species, these alleles disrupt the production of *KIT* receptors, and hence the migration and maturation of melanocytes.

PAX3 belongs to another highly conserved family of transcription factors required for the development of multiple tissue types. It has been shown to act as both a transcriptional activator and a repressor by binding with different proteins. *PAX3* also regulates the genes involved in melanocyte development, one of which is *MITF*, as well as genes involved in pigment synthesis (among others).

Breeds

The American Quarter Horse, Paint horse, Icelandic horse, Shetland pony, Miniature horse, Shire, Clydesdale, Gypsy Vanner, and Welsh pony all exhibit patterns described as splashed white. The *MITF-prom1* allele appears to be distributed among diverse breeds and may have an ancient origin. This allele was found in 58 American Quarter Horses and Paint horses, 11 Icelandic horses, a Shetland pony, and a Miniature horse. The other three mutations appear to be of more recent origin.

Pedigree studies have indicated that *PAX3-C70Y* (*SW2*) originated in a Quarter Horse mare born in 1987. As such, the allele is unlikely to be found in breeds unrelated to the Quarter Horse. *MITF-C280Sfs*20(SW3)* appears to be very rare and possibly restricted to Quarter Horses. *MITF-Macchiato* was a spontaneous mutation found in a Franche-Montagne horse, and is probably unique in the world to that individual, especially as the mutation may have caused the sterility of that horse.

Health concerns

Deafness, only rarely identified in horses, may also be occasionally associated with splashed white, especially in horses that are mostly white, but much more work is needed to substantiate the anecdotal reports of deafness in overos, and to determine the incidence of hearing loss and whether it is associated with a specific white pattern.

Waardenburg's syndrome, another human disease with a distinctive pigment distribution (white forelock) is associated with deafness, and one form of this syndrome has been mapped to the human homolog on chromosome 2 of the mouse *PAX3* gene

(Baldwin *et al.*, 1992). The mouse spotting pattern trait splotch is also assigned to the *PAX3* locus. Another form of Waardenburg's syndrome is on human HSA3, at a site homologous to the mouse microphthalmia (*mi*) gene, associated with white spotting and hearing loss (Tassabehji *et al.*, 1994). Deafness is also associated with white color or spotting patterns in cats, Dalmatians and dogs homozygous for the merle pattern.

References

Baldwin, C.T., Hoth, C.F., Amos, J.A., da-Silva, E.O. and Milunsky, A. (1992) An exonic mutation in the *HUP2* paired domain gene causes Waardenburg's syndrome. *Nature* 355, 637–638.

Dyke, T.M., Laing, E.A. and Hutchins, D.R. (1990) Megacolon in two related Clydesdale foals. *Australian Veterinary Journal* 67, 463–464.

Hauswirth, R. *et al.* (2012) Mutations in *MITF* and *PAX3* cause "splashed white" and other white spotting phenotypes in horses. *PLoS Genetics* 8(4): e1002653, doi:10.1371/journal.pgen.1002653.

Hultgren, B.D. (1982) Ileocolonic aganglionosis in white progeny of overo spotted horses. *Journal of the American Veterinary Medical Association* 180, 289–292.

Klemola, V. (1933) The "pied" and "splashed white" patterns in horses and ponies. *Journal of Heredity* 24, 65–69.

Lightbody, T. (2002) Foal with Overo lethal white syndrome born to a registered quarter horse mare. *Canadian Veterinary Journal* 43, 715–717.

Metallinos, D.L., Bowling, A.T. and Rine, J. (1998) A missense mutation in the endothelin-β receptor gene is associated with lethal white foal syndrome: an equine version of Hirschsprung disease. *Mammalian Genome* 9, 426–431.

Murray, M.J., Parker, G.A. and White, N.A. (1988) Megacolon with myenteric hypoganglionosis in a foal. *Journal of the American Veterinary Medical Association* 192, 917–919.

Puffenberger, E.G., Kauffman, E.R., Bolk, S., Matise, T.C., Washington, S.S., Angrist, M., Weissenbach, J., Garver, K.L., Mascari, M., Ladda, R., Siaugenhaupt, S.A. and Chakravarti, A. (1994) Identity-by-descent and association mapping of a recessive gene for Hirschsprung disease on human chromosome 13q22. *Human Molecular Genetics* 3, 1217–1225.

Santschi, E.M., Purdy, A.K., Valberg, S.J., Vrotsos, P.D., Kaese, H. and Mickelson, J.R. (1998) Endothelin receptor B polymorphism associated with lethal white foal syndrome in horses. *Mammalian Genome* 9, 306–309.

Smith, A.T. (1977) Lethal white foals in mating of overo spotted horses. *Theriogenology* 8, 303–312.

Sponenberg, D.P. (2009) *Equine Color Genetics*, 3rd edn. Wiley-Blackwell, Ames, Iowa.

Tassabehji, M., Newton, V.E. and Read, A.P. (1994) Waardenburg syndrome type 2 caused by mutations in the human microphthalmia (*MITF*)gene. *Nature Genetics* 8, 251–255.

Vonderfecht, S.L., Bowling, A.T. and Cohen, M. (1983) Congenital intestinal aganglionosis in white foals. *Veterinary Pathology* 20, 65–70.

Yang, G.C., Croaker, D., Zhang, A.L., Manglick, P., Cartmill, T. and Cass, D. (1998) A dinucleotide mutation in the endothelin-B receptor gene is associated with lethal white foal syndrome (LWFS); a horse variant of Hirschsprung disease. *Human Molecular Genetics* 7, 1047–1052.

9 Leopard (Appaloosa) Spotting

Leopard Spotting

Leopard complex spotting is the name for the spotting pattern of the Appaloosa horses of the USA, Knabstruppers of Denmark, Norikers of Austria, and many pony breeds from around the world. The pattern is named after one of the distinctive patterns, called "leopard", that is produced by the *Leopard Complex* gene (*LP*). The leopard pattern is composed of dark, oval spots on a white background which extends to cover most of the entire horse. Plate 16 shows an image of a horse with the leopard pattern.

The diversity of phenotypes associated with the *LP* gene is quite extensive and this is why it has been termed the leopard complex. The spotting patterns can range from a sprinkling of a few white hairs on the rump to an almost completely white coat. The patterns go by such names as white specks on the rump, lace blanket, spotted blanket, snow cap blanket, leopard, and "fewspot leopard" (Bellone *et al.*, 2008); some of these are illustrated in Plates 17–19. In general, the patterns are associated with the white distributed symmetrically and centered over the hips, and dark spots of pigment can occur in these white areas. These dark spots are called leopard spots. In addition, horses with the leopard complex trait will show progressive roaning, called varnish roaning (Plate 17), as they age, and the extent of roaning varies from horse to horse. Some of the patterns might be confused with other patterns, especially sabino or roan, except that roaning occurring as a result of the leopard complex will not affect pigment on the bony surfaces of the face, hips, and lower legs. In addition, horses with the trait also exhibit the following additional traits, called "characteristics": striped hooves, unpigmented sclera around the eye, and mottled pigmentation around the anus, genitalia, and muzzle (Sponenberg, 2009).

The Appaloosa horses are a famous color breed originating with the Nez Perce Native Americans of the American Northwest. The name of Appaloosa comes from their origin on the Palouse River of Idaho and Washington. The extent and popularity of the breed has led to the popular use of Appaloosa to describe the leopard complex coat color pattern. However, as noted above, the pattern has a worldwide distribution and may be ancient, having occurred among horses of the Pleistocene period in Europe (Pruvost *et al.*, 2011).

Trait Inheritance and gene symbol

The *Leopard Complex* spotting gene (*LP*) has an incompletely dominant allele (*LP*) which is responsible for the presence of the spotting pattern, in contrast to the recessive allele (*lp*), which is responsible for the absence of *Leopard Complex* spotting. All horses with a single copy of *LP* can exhibit a coat spotting pattern, progressive roaning,

Table 9.1. Genotypes and phenotypes for the *Leopard Complex* (*LP*) gene.

Phenotype	Genotype
Not leopard complex	*lplp*
Leopard complex and characteristics	*LPlp*
Leopard complex with few to no pigmented spots and characteristics, and congenital stationary night blindness (CSNB)	*LPLP*

and the other associated characteristics of *LP*. Horses with two copies of the *LP* allele (*LPLP*) are, however, distinguished by two traits: (i) they have few to no spots of pigment (leopard spots) in the white regions and thus exhibit the patterns called "snowcap blanket" or "fewspot leopard" and (ii) homozygotes for the *LP* allele are affected by congenital stationary night blindness (CSNB), as described below. The phenotypes and genotypes for the Leopard Complex gene are shown in Table 9.1.

The diversity of patterns associated with the appaloosa or leopard patterns initially led to theories that invoked multiple genes to account for the variation in patterns, until Sponenberg *et al.* (1990) convincingly demonstrated that a single major gene with minor gene modifiers was adequate to explain stud book and family data from a variety of breeds. While *LP* is the direct cause of the leopard complex phenotype, the extent of white and the nature of the pattern may be under the control of other, as yet unidentified, genes (Sponenberg, 2009).

Molecular genetics and gene location

Terry *et al.* (2004) investigated the co-segregation of microsatellite DNA markers (see Chapter 11) with genes for appaloosa patterns in several kindred horses (two paternal half-sib families), and found that the genes that were implicated were on ECA1. Within the region implicated on ECA1 the authors noted two genes that might influence pigmentation. The DNA for the protein coding regions of both genes was sequenced without the discovery of a putative *LP* mutation (Bellone *et al.*, 2010a). But when the expression of the two genes was compared in the skin and retina of *LP* and *lp* horses, the expression of the gene for the transient receptor potential cation channel, subfamily M, member 1 (*TRPM1*) was significantly diminished in the skin and retina among horses known to be homozygous for *LP* and affected with CSNB. This suggested that *TRPM1* was responsible for leopard complex spotting, although the mutation responsible for *LP* fell within a region regulating the rate of gene expression that was outside the protein coding portion of the gene. A genetic marker was found useful for predicting whether or not horses had the *LP* gene, but that marker was not the actual mutation (Bellone *et al.*, 2010b; Pruvost *et al.*, 2011). At the time of writing, a manuscript is in preparation that will identify the specific DNA basis for *LP* and CSNB (R.R. Bellone, Tampa, Florida, 2012, personal communication).

Gene function

The product of *TRPM1* belongs to a family of proteins thought to be important for cell migration and signaling through the regulation of calcium ions. *TRPM1*, originally called *Melastatin1*, was selected as a candidate gene because it was inversely expressed in malignant melanoma, thus suggesting a role in normal melanogenesis (Duncan *et al.*, 1998). While its role in melanogenesis is not yet fully elucidated in humans, it has been suggested to be involved in melanin storage (Oancea *et al.*, 2009). Mice and humans with mutations in *TRPM1* have CSNB but no pigmentation differences in these animals have been discovered to date.

Breeds

The pattern is found among many other breeds around the world, including Knabstruppers of Denmark, Norikers of Austria, and many pony breeds from around the world.

Health concerns

CSNB is an inherited condition of horses shown to be completely associated in Appaloosa and American Miniature Horses with homozygosity for the *LP* allele (Sandmeyer *et al.*, 2007, 2012; Bellone *et al.*, 2008). The condition manifests as apparently normal vision in full light but greatly diminished vision under low light conditions. Such horses may appear clumsy or apprehensive when moving around objects when under low light. However, the eyes do not exhibit abnormal morphology, even under microscopic examination. Clinical diagnosis is based on electroretinography examination by veterinary ophthalmologists (Sandmeyer *et al.*, 2007, 2012). *TRPM1* controls polarization of the on-bipolar cell, which is the cell responsible for transmitting the signal from the rod photoreceptor cell in the eye under low light conditions. Thus, the causative mutation in leopard pattern horses is thought to affect *TRPM1* signaling (R.R. Bellone, Tampa, Florida, 2012, personal communication). Horses with one copy of the *LP* allele appear to be unaffected. Owners are often surprised to learn that their horses have CSNB, despite years of working with them. Horses have excellent memories and learn to compensate for poor night vision, both by following the herd when moving at night or by memorizing the location of objects in paddocks or stalls. To protect these animals, safe fencing should be used; affected horses should also be kept with pasture mates at night, or in well light paddocks or stalls; and caution should be exercised when entering a dark barn or trailer.

References

Bellone, R.R., Brooks, S.A., Sandmeyer, L., Murphy, B.A., Forsyth, G., Archer, S., Bailey, E. and Grahn, B. (2008) Differential gene expression of *TRPM1*, the potential cause of congenital stationary night blindness and coat spotting patterns (*LP*) in Appaloosa horses (*Equus caballus*). *Genetics* 179, 1861–1870.

Bellone, R.R. *et al.* (2010a) Fine-mapping and mutation analysis of *TRPM*: a candidate gene for leopard complex (*LP*) spotting and congenital stationary night blindness in horses. *Briefings in Functional Genomics* 9, 193–207.

Bellone, R.R., Archer, S., Wade, C.M., Cuka-Lawson, C., Haase, B., Leeb, T., Forsyth, G., Sandmeyer, L. and Grahn, B. (2010b) Association analysis of candidate SNPs in *TRPM1* with leopard complex spotting (*LP*) and congenital stationary night blindness (CSNB) in horses. *Animal Genetics* 42 (Supplement 2), 207.

Duncan, L.M., Deeds, J., Hunter, J., Shao, J., Holmgren, L.M., Woolf, E.A., Tepper, R.I. and Shyjan, A.W. (1998) Down-regulation of the novel gene melastatin correlates with potential for melanoma metastasis. *Cancer Research* 58, 1515–1520.

Oancea, E., Vriens, J., Brauchi, S., Jun, J., Splawski, I. and Clapham, D.E. (2009) *TRPM1* forms ion channels associated with melanin content in melanocytes. *Science Signaling* 2(70), ra21.

Pruvost, M., Bellone, R., Benecke, N., Sandoval-Castellanos, E., Cieslak, M., Kuznetsova, T., Morales-Muñiz, A., O'Connor, T., Reissmann, M., Hofreiter, M. and Ludwig, A. (2011) Genotypes of predomestic horses match phenotypes painted in Paleolithic works of cave art. *Proceedings of the National Academy of Sciences of the United States of America* 108, 18626–18630.

Sandmeyer, L.S., Breaux, C.B., Archer, S. and Grahn, B.H. (2007) Clinical and electroretinographic characteristics of congenital stationary night blindness in the Appaloosa and the association with the leopard complex. *Veterinary Ophthalmology* 10, 368–375.

Sandmeyer, L.S., Bellone, R.R., Archer, S., Bauer, B.S., Nelson, J., Forsyth, G. and Grahn, B.H. (2012) Congenital stationary night blindness is associated with the leopard complex in the miniature horse. *Veterinary Ophthalmology* 15, 18–22.

Sponenberg, D.P. (2009) *Equine Color Genetics*, 3rd edn. Wiley-Blackwell, Ames, Iowa.

Sponenberg, D.P., Carr, G., Simak, E. and Schwink, K. (1990) The inheritance of the leopard complex of spotting patterns in horses. *Journal of Heredity* 81, 323–331.

Terry, R.B., Archer, S., Brooks, S., Bernoco, D. and Bailey, E. (2004) Assignment of the appaloosa coat colour gene (*LP*) to equine chromosome 1. *Animal Genetics* 35, 134–137.

10 Putting It All Together: Color by Design

Horse breeders understood the genetics of coat color long before DNA tests were developed. The thought occurs: "The color of a horse is apparent just by looking at it. Why do we need DNA tests?" Actually, there are several specific applications for these tests:

1. Horses homozygous for a gene will always transmit the gene to its offspring. This has been particularly useful for breeders of tobiano horses. Tobiano horses usually look the same, whether they have one or two copies of the gene. Genetic tests can quickly determine the likelihood of producing tobiano offspring from a mating by determining whether the horse has one or two copies of *TO* of the *TO* allele.

2. Some color patterns look similar despite distinctive genetic origins. While some experts can distinguish cream dilution and champagne dilution, the DNA test is definitive. The overo, sabino, dominant white, and other spotting patterns also can be difficult to distinguish. We do not have tests for all spotting patterns, but we can certainly make exclusions or inclusions using the existing tests.

3. Gray will mask the underlying coat color. Genetic tests can determine the potential of a gray horse to produce chestnut, black, bay, diluted, tobiano, or leopard patterns with the use of molecular genetic tests.

4. Identification of the molecular basis of a trait will help us to understand the nature of some associated hereditary diseases, such as overo lethal white (foal) syndrome (OLWS), homozygous lethal white or homozygous lethal roan, the association of melanoma with gray, deafness associated with splashed white, and congenital stationary night blindness (CSNB) associated with the leopard complex.

5. Identification of the genes responsible for the different patterns will help to identify other genes that modify those patterns. Considerable work is underway to identify modifiers of the *Leopard Complex* gene (Sponenberg, 2009). We have not yet identified modifiers of the *Extension* gene leading to the variants popularly referred to as light sorrel, liver chestnut, or brown.

The preceding chapters are limited in their discussion of coat colors in horses. Other books and some of the online media do a much better job of describing the diversity of color patterns (Sponenberg, 2009, for example). Our chapters have focused on the remarkable, but limited, contributions of molecular genetics to the understanding of hair color in horses. This information is summarized in Table 10.1. For example, we now know that dominant white is the product of not one, but many different mutations. We know that sabino, tobiano, dominant white and roan are related to each other as different mutations of the same gene (*KIT*). We know that sabino has more than one genetic cause (*SB1*) because the *SB1* locus is not responsible

Table 10.1. Color genes for horses.

Locus name	Effect on coat color	Locus symbol	Gene	Alleles	Mutation	Mode of inheritance	Associated disease
Agouti (bay)	Restrict black pigment to points	A	ASIP	A a	Wild type Missense	Dominant Recessive	None None
Appaloosa	White spotting plus leopard complex (LP) characteristics	LP	TRPM1	lp LP	Wild type Not reported	Recessive Incomplete dominant	None Homozygous CSNB,[a] susceptibility to uveitis
Champagne Dilution	Dilution of black and red pigment	CH	SLC36A	ch CH	Wild type Missense	Recessive Incomplete dominant	None None
Cream Dilution	Dilution of red pigment	CR	SLC45A2	cr CR	Wild type Missense	Recessive Incomplete dominant	None None
				pr	Not reported	–	–
Dominant White	White spotting	W	KIT	w W1–W17	Wild type See Table 6.2	Recessive Incomplete dominant	None Some homozygous lethal
Dun	Dilution with black points and back stripe	D	Unknown	d D	Wild type Unknown	Recessive Dominant	None None
Extension (black and chestnut)	Black and red pigment	E	MC1R	E e	Wild type Missense	Dominant Recessive	None None
Frame Overo	White spotting	O	EDNRB	o O	Wild type Missense	Recessive Incomplete dominant	None Homozygous OLWS[b]
Gray	Loss of hair pigment with age	G	STX17	g G	Wild type Gene duplication	Recessive Dominant	None Susceptibility to melanoma

Trait	Description	Symbol	Gene	Allele	Mutation	Inheritance	Health
Roan	Roaning	RN	KIT	rn	Wild type	Recessive	None
				RN	Unknown	Incomplete dominant	Some homozygous lethal
Sabino1	White spotting	SB1	KIT	sb1	Wild type	Recessive	None
				SB1	Splice variant	Incomplete dominant	None
Silver Dilution	Dilution of black pigment	Z	PMEL17	z	Wild type	Recessive	None
				Z	Missense	Incomplete dominant	None
Splashed White (MITF)	White spotting	MITF	MITF	MITF+	Wild type	Recessive	None
				MITF-prom1	Insertion	Dominant	None
				MITF-C280Sfs*20	Deletion	Dominant	Possible homozygous lethal
				MITF-N310S	Missense	Dominant	Possible homozygous lethal
Splashed White (PAX3)	White spotting	PAX3	PAX3	PAX3+	Wild type	Recessive	None
				PAX3-C70Y	Missense	Dominant	Possible homozygous lethal
Tobiano	White spotting	TO	KIT	to	Wild type	Recessive	None
				TO	Inversion	Dominant	None

[a]CSNB, congenital stationary night blindness.
[b]OLWS, overo lethal white syndrome.

for the sabino pattern seen in Clydesdale horses. We know that depigmentation caused by the *Overo*, *Splashed White*, *Leopard*, and *Gray* loci are all products of other genes.

We do not know the genetic basis for modifiers of *Extension* or *Leopard*. We do not know the genetic basis of sabino in Clydesdale horses. The genetic causes remain unknown for brindle, Birdcatcher spots, a flaxen mane and tail, dappling and white markings on the face and leg. We do not know what causes variation in the extent or distribution of white spotting for the tobiano, overo or any of the other spotting phenotypes. However, we have reason to believe that this ignorance is temporary. The genomic tools used to identify the loci described in these chapters are clearly adequate for characterizing the genes responsible for these and other simple hereditary traits in horses. Indeed, the largest challenge to solving these questions is in accurately identifying color patterns and assembling the correct group of horses for investigation. Consider this: if the investigations of sabino had combined data from Tennessee Walking Horses and Clydesdales, the *SB1* locus would never have been identified. If horses with the tobiano, splashed white, and frame overo patterns had been combined to discover a common gene for white patterns, the study would have failed. The observations, experience and wisdom of breeders are key to designing the right questions for research.

The studies that have been carried out have demonstrated two other important points.

- Firstly, the color of horses matters. Archeological studies and molecular data suggest that people selected horses for the diversity of their color patterns (Ludwig *et al.*, 2009). Before domestication, molecular tests suggest that horses were predominantly dark colored. The genes for white patterns and dilutions appeared after domestication. Early people must have taken pride in the appearance of their horses, as well as in their ability and willingness to work.
- Second, the genes that influence coat color patterns in one species often play a similar role in another. The *MC1R* gene encodes the alleles for red and black of the *Extension* locus in horses, humans, cattle, dogs, and other species. Mutations in the gene *KIT* cause various types of white spotting in horses (tobiano, roan, sabino, dominant white), mice, and humans. The gene for overo in horses was discovered because of its homology to a white hair gene seen for human Hirschprung's disease (*EDNRB*). Molecular studies demonstrated that it was true in many cases that the genes that influence coat color patterns in one species often play a similar role in another. It was not a surprise. Based simply on phenotype, earlier geneticists assumed that coat colors in horses were due to the action of gene homologous to those found in other species (Castle, 1948). This is an important lesson for genetic studies: we can use the lessons learned in other species.

Finally, the appearance of novel colors, especially those associated with white spotting, is a hallmark of domestication (Cieslak *et al.*, 2011). Certainly, this is in part due to the release of natural selection against conspicuous, poorly camouflaged patterns associated with pleiotropic health defects. However, as pathways influencing both behavior and color involve cells that originate at the embryonic neural crest, the concurrent acquisition of tame behaviour and novel coat colors may not be coincidental. The study of coat color patterns in the horse is a study of the nature of the horse.

References

Castle, W.E. (1948) The ABC of color inheritance in the horse. *Genetics* 33, 22–35.

Cieslak, M., Reissmann, M., Hofreiter, M. and Ludwig, A. (2011) Colours of domestication. *Biological Reviews* 86, 885–899.

Ludwig, A., Pruvost, M., Reissmann, M., Benecke, N., Brockmann, G.A., Castanos, P., Cieslak, M., Lippold, S., Llorente, L., Malaspinas, A.S., Slatkin, M. and Hofreiter, M. (2009) Coat color variation at the beginning of horse domestication. *Science* 324, 485.

Sponenberg, D.P. (2009) *Equine Color Genetics*, 3rd edn. Wiley-Blackwell, Ames, Iowa.

11 Parentage Testing

Parentage

Many of the traits we value in horses are highly heritable. Breeders have long known that offspring tend to resemble their parents. Consequently, pedigrees and parentage are important. Most horse breed registries have instituted rules that require some form of genetic testing to verify the parentage of registered horses. This chapter explains the genetics of parentage testing.

Two rules of parentage testing

Parentage testing is based on two simple rules:

1. Every genetic factor (allele) present in a foal must be present in at least one of the parents.
2. The parents must contribute one genetic factor (allele) from each of their genes to the foal.

Of course, these rules pertain to genes found on autosomes. Special cases may arise with respect to genes on sex chromosomes and mitochondria, and these will be discussed later.

Rule 1 has long been known and applied by horse breeders in connection with coat color inheritance. One application was the "Gray Rule". The gray coat color pattern is the result of a dominant gene. If a foal has the *Gray* gene, then one of its parents must also possess the *Gray* gene. Another example of coat colors applied to rule 1 is the "Chestnut Rule". When both parents are chestnut, they cannot have a foal that is black or bay. Chestnut horses lack the dominant gene for black hair pigment; accordingly, at least one parent of a black or bay foal must have black hair.

Rule 2 is dependent upon the use of codominant genetic traits, and upon the use of the genetic markers such as blood groups, biochemical markers, or DNA markers, which are described below. Indeed, the development of genetic makers made it easy to apply rules 1 and 2 to parentage testing. However, this brings us to the consequences and limitations of parentage testing.

Parentage testing detects errors in pedigrees but does not prove parentage

Our two rules for parentage testing determine when a foal does not belong to two parents according to genetic tests. If the rules are violated, we know that the stated parentage is incorrect. So be aware, parentage testing excludes incorrect parents, *but it does not prove parentage*! There is no scientific way to prove parentage as such. But if we do enough tests, the chance of having an incorrect parentage and passing all the tests becomes diminishingly small. At that point, we consider that the stated mating qualifies for parentage.

These points will be easier to understand by way of example. First though, we must consider the types of genetic tests that have been used for parentage testing. In the 1960s, blood typing (described below) was developed and used for parentage testing. In the 1990s, DNA testing was implemented, and has almost completely replaced blood typing as the method of choice.

Blood typing tests

The first genetic factors used for parentage testing were blood group factors. Blood groups in horses are analogous to those in humans, for instance the ABO and RH systems. Blood groups are proteins or carbohydrates on the surface of blood cells which can be readily detected in laboratory tests. However, human blood typing reagents did not work on horses, and scientists needed to make new reagents to discover horse blood groups. Ultimately, eight genetic systems were uncovered with at least 34 factors that exhibited a codominant mode of inheritance, and were inherited equally from stallions and mares (these are reviewed in Sandberg and Cothran, 2000). Scientists also investigated proteins and enzymes in blood to uncover genetic variants. Here, they discovered 16 genetic systems with at least 82 factors, again, each exhibiting a codominant mode of inheritance, and equal inheritance from sire and dam (also reviewed in Sandberg and Cothran, 2000). Beginning in the 1960s, laboratories began using these genetic tests for parentage testing. Typically, the laboratories would choose 12–15 of these genetic systems for routine testing. As mentioned above, this approach to parentage testing has now been almost entirely replaced by DNA techniques, which is described in the next section.

DNA Tests

Obviously, DNA is a great target for parentage testing. After all, it is the molecule of heredity. Variation seen in blood groups, enzymes, proteins, and coat color merely reflects differences in DNA molecules. But before the scientific advances in the 1990s, we did not have a good way to test DNA. Inventions associated with the human genome project and research on horses led to the development of inexpensive, powerful and rapid methods for testing DNA and conducting parentage tests. At the same time, the development of this new testing method was not the only important consideration in changing from blood typing to DNA typing.

A major driver for the change to DNA testing was the reduced costs and effort needed for collecting, shipping, and saving samples. DNA tests do not require blood samples. DNA can be extracted from any tissue (including blood). Consequently, methods were developed to extract DNA from horse's hair or from buccal swabs. As horse owners were competent in plucking hairs or collecting buccal swabs, the adoption of DNA testing for parentage could ease the process, and reduce the costs of sample collection. Furthermore, hairs and buccal swabs were more robust than blood samples for shipping and unlikely to spoil. Indeed, hair samples could be saved without freezing or refrigeration for years before testing.

As noted in Chapter 3, the genome of the horse is complex. Among the 2.49 billion bases of DNA, mutations have occurred that have resulted in detectable, hereditary differences between horses. To be effective for parentage testing, the genetic differences needed to be detected with high accuracy, and to be inexpensive, repeatable, and rapidly testable. In the 1990s, several types of DNA variants were considered. The type of genetic difference that was found to be most useful for parentage testing in horses was a type of genetic marker called a microsatellite DNA. Other names for this type of genetic variant have been short tandem repeat (STR), variable number of tandem repeats (VNTRs) and trinucleotide or dinucleotide repeats. Here, we will use the term microsatellite.

Microsatellite DNA markers

Microsatellite DNA markers are short stretches of DNA that exhibit a serial repetition of a pair of DNA bases. They are also known as simple sequence repeats (SSRs) or short tandem repeats (STRs), and are a type of variable number tandem repeat (VNTR) (see Chapter 10). For example, "TGTGTGTGTGTGTGTGTGTGTGTG" is a representation of such a series on one strand of the DNA molecule; it could also be represented as (TG)12, denoting a series of 12 iterations of TG. These repeats do not occur in the genes themselves, but rather in intergenic DNA. Another characteristic of these sequences is that they tend to have extensive genetic variation when compared between horses.

An example of a microsatellite DNA marker found at a specific spot on horse chromosome 15 (ECA15) is HTG6 (Marklund *et al.*, 1994). The number of repeats found in HTG6 for different strands of ECA15 varied from 20, i.e. (TG)20, to 12, i.e. (TG)12. For unknown reasons, the higher the number of repeats in a microsatellite, the more likely it will show variation between chromosomes. Molecular genetic studies in several species have indicated that more than 100,000 microsatellites exist with more than 12 repeats of dinucleotides. During the 1990s, scientists discovered many microsatellite DNA markers that are suitable for use in DNA parentage tests for horses.

Testing microsatellites

Several different approaches have been used for testing microsatellites, but they do have some common aspects. The main point is that the HTG6 marker represented by (TG)20 is longer than the HTG6 marker represented by (TG)12 by eight nucleotides. For genetic tests of HTG6, we just need to measure the differences in the length of the HTG6 segment on each of the two chromosomes in each horse. Believe it or not, this can be done simply.

Polymerase chain reaction (PCR)

As noted above, the "TG" repeats characteristic of microsatellites, including HTG6, are very common, with about 100,000 in the genome. However, the regions surrounding the TG repeats are unique to that place in the genome. So, to define HTG6, scientists use the 200–300 bases surrounding the TG repeat. Nowhere else in the genome are there DNA sequences that are the same as those in the HGT6 segment. Then again, 200–300 DNA bases are miniscule compared with the 2,490,000,000 bases in the genome. Finding the 200–300 DNA bases for HTG6 in the entire genome is akin to finding a needle in a haystack. The solution is to use PCR. We place a small amount of total DNA from a horse in a test tube. This is the haystack. The PCR reaction involves the use of two fragments of DNA, called primers or probes, which seek out and bind to the genomic DNA on either side of HTG6. This is the needle. Then an enzyme that replicates DNA (commonly, Taq polymerase) is used to make a copy of the DNA between the two primers. The process is typically repeated 30 times, and each time the amount of HTG6 DNA is doubled. While this does not seem like much initially, at the end of 30 cycles of replication, there are millions of copies of the HTG6 DNA. With reference to our haystack analogy, there is so much DNA that the original haystack has become buried under a pile of needles.

Measuring the length of a microsatellite

As noted above, the genetic variation detectable for HTG6 is apparent as differences in the length of the molecule. DNA molecules have an electrical charge, and we can cause them to move by applying an electric current. If we make a gel matrix with holes that allow smaller molecules to move faster, then we can separate large molecules from small molecules. This is precisely the basis of current tests. The gels used by horse parentage testing laboratories are designed to resolve DNA molecules that differ by a single DNA base. They are subjected to an electric current for a certain period of time. The DNA is labeled with one of many possible dyes and the sizes of the DNA fragments are measured.

Our example focused on the microsatellite marker HTG6. This same process is used for another 11–15 microsatellite DNA markers that are used in routine tests. The tests can be automated, and the results recorded on a computer as a simple measure for the size of the microsatellite allele.

International Collaboration and Oversight of Horse Parentage Testing

Many laboratories provide parentage testing for horses. When horses are shipped around the world it becomes important for each laboratory to be able to read the parentage testing reports from other laboratories. To do so, it is important that the laboratories test for the same genetic markers and use the same nomenclature. This standardization is achieved through a voluntary collaboration among the scientists that provide this service. Every 2 years scientists performing horse parentage testing participate in a standardization test conducted under the auspices of the International Society of Animal Genetics.

International Society of Animal Genetics (ISAG)

The society originally began as a loose confederation of scientists working on genetic markers in animals. Its first conference was held in 1954. In the period from the 1940s to the 1960s, genetic markers were discovered for horses and other animals by testing for blood groups or for blood proteins. Comparison tests began in the 1962 for cattle, and at this stage scientists began meeting on a biannual basis to compare genetic variants and to standardize the nomenclature. Later, comparison tests were added for horses and other species. The scientists overseeing these comparison tests and conferences formed a scientific society, initially called the European Society of Animal Blood Groups and Biochemical Genetics. Later, in 1972, the name of the society was changed to the International Society of Animal Blood Groups and Biochemical Genetics, so as to reflect membership from the Americas, Australasian regions, and Africa. In 1988, the name was changed to the International Society of Animal Genetics to reflect the broad interests of the society's scientists in understanding the genetics of domestic animals. More information about the ISAG can be found at their website (see Website section at end of chapter for URL).

ISAG comparison tests

All scientists providing parentage testing service in horses participate in the biannual comparison test. When the test was based on blood typing, blood samples were provided to each laboratory, and each would test the samples for genetic variants they could recognize. Much research was done to discover new genetic systems, and this was a means for the laboratories to collaborate on their discoveries. When two or more laboratories identified the same genetic variants in two subsequent comparison tests, the ISAG committee would assign official nomenclature for the marker. Collaboration was very important when specific blood group reagents needed to be made, or when specific recipes needed to be followed to evaluate blood proteins.

In the 1990s, DNA replaced blood groups and biochemical markers for parentage testing for the reasons that have already been stated. The ISAG comparison tests are still conducted on a biannual basis, but with the goal of standardizing the recognition of genetic markers. Because horses are shipped internationally, coordination among laboratories is important at the international level. At the 2010 ISAG horse parentage testing workshop, the laboratories agreed to test the following microsatellite markers for the parentage testing of horses: AHT4, AHT5, ASB17, ASB2, ASB23, HMS2, HMS3, HMS6, HMS7, HTG10, HTG4, and VHL20. These markers provide sufficient power to identify horses and to resolve most questions of parentage. However, most laboratories also test for additional markers to resolve disputed parentage, or to address special needs for the horse populations under study.

Example of a Parentage Case Using Microsatellite DNA Markers

Table 11.1 shows an example of a parentage case designed to identify which of two stallions is the correct sire of a foal. The table shows the results of tests for eight

Table 11.1. Horse parentage case resolved using microsatellite DNA markers.

Horse	Microsatellite locus and alleles					
	AHT4	*AHT5*	*HTG4*	*HTG6*	*VHL20*	*LEX003*
Stallion 1	*LQ*	*MO*	*NQ*	*LP*	*NO*	*P*
Stallion 2	*LM*	*NO*	*NP*	*KL*	*PO*	*P*
Dam	*KQ*	*MO*	*MO*	*KP*	*NP*	*KS*
Offspring	*KM*	*MO*	*MP*	*KL*	*NO*	*KP*

microsatellite loci. At the ISAG conferences, the horse parentage testing laboratories compare their results for testing each microsatellite on the same group of horses. Based on the consistency of their typing results on the entire panel of tests, the laboratories assign letter names to each of the microsatellite alleles. So, for the *AHT4* locus, stallion 1 is heterozygous for the *L* and *Q* alleles. Stallion 2 is heterozygous for the *L* and *M* alleles. Every laboratory in the world that does parentage testing on horses and participates in the ISAG comparison test will agree on that. We can use these markers to apply rules 1 and 2 to determine which of the two stallions is the correct sire of the offspring.

1. For the *AHT4* locus, the offspring possesses the *K* and *M* alleles. The *K* allele could have come from the dam, so *M* must have come from the sire. Only Stallion 2 has the *M* allele, so stallion 1 is excluded.
2. For the *AHT5* locus, the offspring possesses *M* and *O*. The dam has both. The sires must possess one of them. Sire 1 possesses both. Sire 2 possesses *O*, so both qualify as parents based on the *AHT5* locus.
3. For the *HTG4* locus, the offspring possesses *M* and *P*. The dam possesses *M* so the sire must possess *P*. Only Stallion 2 possesses *P*, so Stallion 2 qualifies, while Stallion 1 is excluded.
4. For the *HTG6* locus, the offspring possesses *K* and *L*, of which the dam only possesses *K*, so *L* must come from the sire. Both stallions possess *L*, and so both qualify as parents based on the *HTG6* locus.
5. For the *VHL20* locus, the offspring possesses *N* and *O*, while the dam only possesses *O*, so the *O* allele must have come from the sire. Both stallions have the *O* allele and, therefore, neither is excluded on the basis of the *VHL20* locus.
6. For the *LEX003* locus, the offspring has alleles *K* and *P*. The dam only has *K* so *P* must come from the sire. Both sires have *P*, and so they are not excluded on the basis of the *LEX003* locus. Note that LEX003 is a special marker because it is found on the X chromosome. As you may recall from Chapter 2, mares have two X chromosomes while stallions have only one. For this reason, stallions will only have one allele for the *LEX003* locus while females may have two. In this case, we can see that the stallions have one allele and the dam has two. We can also see that the offspring has two alleles for the X chromosome and is female.

In summary, Stallion 1 is excluded as the sire on the basis of test results for the *AHT4* and *HTG4* microsatellite loci; Stallion 2 qualified at all loci and could be the correct sire; finally, the results from the *LEX003* locus show that the offspring is female.

Special cases

Usually, two horses will have different genetic types, and these genetic tests can distinguish between them, and exclude incorrectly assigned parents. However, the following situations require special attention:

1. Identical twins. Identical twins occur on very rare occasions when a fertilized egg splits to form two embryos. These twins are also called monozygotic twins. Identical twins have identical genetic markers. Specifically, they will test the same in practically all genetic tests. The only differences between twins are rare mutations that occur in germ line cells during development, and aspects of development that are not entirely genetic. For example, identical human twins have different fingerprints. Identical twin horses will have similar but not identical hair whorls and white pattern distributions. The standard microsatellite DNA tests are unlikely to distinguish between identical twins, and, consequently, are unlikely to distinguish between twins as the parent of a foal. Of course, genetically, it should not make any difference. Identical twins will be identical in the opportunities afforded by the genes that they transmit to offspring.

2. Fraternal twins. Fraternal twins occur when a female produces two eggs and each is fertilized by a different sperm. Even though the foals are carried in the womb simultaneously, they are genetically related only as full siblings. Existing genetic tests have sufficient power to distinguish between them as possible parents for a foal.

3. Cloning by splitting embryos. Cloning is the production of individuals with identical genetic characteristics. One way to produce clones is to isolate an early embryo and split it to produce two or more additional embryos. The products of split embryos are clones and identical to the identical twins that are described above. In this case, there is no way to distinguish between potential parents that are clones and, as in identical twins, there is no difference in genetic contribution possible from clones of the same embryo.

4. Clones by nuclear transfer. In recent years, it has become possible to transfer the nucleus of one mature horse into an enucleated egg and produce an embryo with the genes of the mature horse. Clones produced in this way will have identical genetic markers as determined by the nucleus of the mature horse. This includes all of the genetic markers that are currently tested by parentage testing laboratories. However, the nuclear transfer does not replace the mitochondrial DNA of the egg. Clones produced by nuclear transfer will have the mitochondrial DNA of the enucleated egg. DNA tests of mitochondria may distinguish between nuclear transfer cloned mares because they transmit mitochondria to their offspring. But this will only work when the eggs for cloning come from different, unrelated donor mares. Stallions do not transfer their mitochondria to offspring, so a mitochondrial DNA test will not make that distinction.

5. Blood chimeras. On rare occasions, twin foals will share a blood supply during early embryogenesis. When this occurs, stem cells from the blood-producing cells of one twin may become implanted within the body of the other twin. As a consequence, that other twin will produce the blood cells of its own genetic type as well as the blood cells of the twin. This may become an issue with fraternal twins. It is possible for the blood cells of the twin to completely replace the blood cells of the individual. In this case, tests of blood cells will detect genes different from the genes in the

germinal tissue, testes, and ovaries. When this happens, the blood type of the parent will not be compatible with the parentage of its offspring (Bowling *et al.*, 1993). Fortunately, this can be readily detected by testing DNA from a tissue biopsy, such as skin. Tissues other than blood will be found to match the DNA type of the germinal tissue.

Future Applications of Genetic Testing for Parentage and Identity

The power of genetic testing to address questions of parentage and identity depends on the number of tests run. Currently, hundreds of alleles are evaluated using the microsatellite tests. The genome projects have invented more powerful tools as well, but these are not necessarily better for application to parentage and identity. For example, scientists use a tool called the SNP chip (SNPs are discussed in Chapter 3), which employs 70,000 out of the 1.47 million known genetic variants for horses. This tool would be very powerful for parentage and identity purposes, though the cost would be prohibitive. At the time of writing, the cost of running the SNP chip test is about US$200, while the cost of doing microsatellite testing is below US$30. There are two issues that drive the choice of parentage test for horses: (i) the cost of running the test; and (ii) the ability to use the genetic information that has been derived from previous tests. To do a parentage analysis, the genetic results from the parents and the offspring must be available. Currently, microsatellite results are stored in an extensive computerized database, and it is these records that are used in parentage analysis. So once a horse has been tested, it need not be tested again. Only if a new type of test is to be used will all horses need to be retested.

Horse breeders encountered this problem when they switched parentage testing from blood typing to microsatellite testing. The costs of the tests were very similar. The power of the tests was also similar, but to test DNA, one did not need a blood sample. DNA could be extracted from hair follicles or buccal swabs. While blood samples were often collected by veterinarians, hair and buccal swabs could be collected by horse owners. While blood samples needed to be shipped by express mail services to avoid spoilage, DNA in hair and buccal swabs was stable and could be shipped by regular mail services. The cost savings for sample processing compelled registries and horse owners to change the methods of testing used. Although horses that had previously been blood typed needed to be retested for DNA, the costs were less in the long term.

What advantage might encourage breeders to change the test method again – to SNP testing? As described in other chapters of this book, many genetic tests have been developed and are commercially available that do use SNP tests. If the use of these tests becomes widespread among horse breeders, then it might become economically advantageous to change to a parentage test based on SNPs, but with added information about coat color genetics, disease genes, and performance genetics.

References

Bowling, A.T., Stott, M.L. and Bickel, L. (1993) Silent blood chimaerism in a mare confirmed by DNA marker analysis of hair bulbs. *Animal Genetics* 24, 323–324.

Marklund, S., Ellegern, H., Eriksson, S., Sandberg, K. and Andersson, L. (1994) Parentage testing and linkage analysis in the horse using a set of highly polymorphic microsatellites. *Animal Genetics* 25, 19–23.

Sandberg, K. and Cothran, E.G. (2000) Biochemical genetics and blood groups. In: Bowling, A.T. and Ruvinsky, A. (eds) *The Genetics of the Horse*. CAB International, Wallingford, pp. 85–108.

Website

International Society of Animal Genetics (ISAG). Available at: http://www.isag.us/ (accessed 10 December 2012).

12 Medical Genetics

Horse breeders justifiably pride themselves on their knowledge of pedigrees, having an eye for conformation, and having an ability to design matings that produce horses that are stronger, faster and more athletic than those of the previous generation. Every foaling is exciting and attached to the question: "How good could this one be?" Health problems seem a distant, though tragic, possibility. When health problems have a hereditary component, the effect is ironic. Hereditary diseases mock the skills of the breeder who has planned things so well. Fortunately, such diseases are uncommon, and breeders will be most effective when they select for performance and not against disease. Nevertheless, astute breeders pay attention to genetic problems as these can prevent an otherwise perfect horse from realizing its potential.

Genetic influences on disease are suspected when a condition is prevalent in some populations but not others, or when the condition shows a familial tendency. Dissecting out the genetic component may be difficult. This chapter describes some of the investigations that have been made into genetic influences on diseases in horses, and is divided into four main sections. These discuss: (i) simple Mendelian hereditary diseases for which there are DNA tests available; (ii) Mendelian disease genes not yet characterized at the DNA level; (iii) complex hereditary diseases and quantitative trait loci (QTLs); and (iv) neonatal isoerythorolysis. To finish the chapter, brief mention is also made of the database Online Mendelian Inheritance in Animals, which includes information on hereditary diseases of the horse.

Cytogenetics is clearly also relevant to veterinary medical genetics, and merits its own chapter: Chapter 13 (The Horse Karyotype and Chromosomal Abnormalities).

Simple Mendelian Hereditary Diseases Characterized at the Molecular Level

Many diseases are the result of a mutation in a single gene, a mutation which can either destroy the function of the gene or create a function which is disruptive. Such mutations are inherited in a Mendelian fashion as simple recessive or dominant traits. If the trait is dominant, its effect is seen immediately in heterozygotes and selection can be applied. This may occur when the mutation causes a new disruptive function for the gene. In those cases, affected offspring will also have affected parents. So breeders need to know the health of their breeding stock.

Recessive mutations present a different story. A single copy of a recessive mutation will not be detectable. If two carriers of a recessive disease mutation are bred, there will be a chance (25%) that the foal will inherit both disease-causing genes. Genetic tests can identify carriers for some diseases, but unless the breeder suspects a carrier and does a test, or if there is no test, the first evidence that a horse carries a gene for a recessive hereditary disease is the production of a foal with that disease.

The following subsections describe some of the simple, Mendelian hereditary diseases that have been characterized at the molecular level (Table 12.1). They are organized by breed, based on the breed in which the disease gene was first found. In some cases, the gene appears to be restricted to that breed. In other cases, the gene can be found among horses of other breeds, thus reflecting the relationship among horse breeds.

Breed: American Quarter Horses

Hyperkalemic periodic paralysis (HYPP)

HYPP is a muscle disease found predominantly among Quarter Horses. Horses with this gene have a well-developed musculature and are often favored in halter classes. Other aspects of the condition include a wide range of symptoms, such as muscle

Table 12.1. Simple Mendelian hereditary diseases of horses for which there are molecular DNA diagnostic tests, with information on the genes responsible, mode of inheritance, and breeds affected.

Disease[a]	Acronym	Gene	Mode of Inheritance	Breeds affected
Hyperkalemic periodic paralysis	HYPP	SCN4A	Dominant	Quarter Horse
Hereditary equine regional dermal asthenia	HERDA	PPIB	Recessive	Quarter Horse
Glycogen branching enzyme deficiency	GBED	GBE1	Recessive	Quarter Horse
Type 1 polysaccharide storage myopathy	PSSM1	GYS1	Dominant	Quarter Horse
Malignant hyperthermia	MH	RYR1	Dominant	Quarter Horse
Severe combined immunodeficiency disease	SCID	DNA-PK	Recessive	Arabian
Lavender foal syndrome	LFS	MYO5A	Recessive	Arabian
Cerebellar abiotrophy	CA	TOE1 or MUTYH	Recessive	Arabian
Junctional epidemolysis bullosa (JEB-LAMC2)	JEB-LAMC2	LAMC2	Recessive	Belgian draft
Junctional epidemolysis bullosa (JEB-LAMC3)	JEB-LAMA3	LAMA3	Recessive	American Saddlebred
Foal immunodeficiency syndrome	FIS	SMIT or SLC5A3	Recessive	Fell and Dale pony
Congenital stationary night blindness	CSNB	TRPM1	Recessive	Appaloosa spotted
Lethal white foal syndrome	LWFS	EDNRB	Recessive	Frame Overo spotted

[a] Diseases are listed in the order in which they are described in the first section of the chapter.

tremors, paralysis, temporary muscle weakness, and collapse. The symptoms are similar to a condition in humans, which led scientists to DNA sequence the homologous gene in horses. HYPP is the result of a mutation in the gene *SCN4A*, which regulates sodium transport in muscles. The mutation changes an amino acid in a critical portion of the coded molecule, the skeletal muscle sodium channel alpha subunit (Rudolph *et al.*, 1992). The specific details of this mutation were provided as an example of DNA mutations in Chapter 2. Under normal conditions, the muscle cell opens sodium channels briefly during activation, but muscle cells with the mutated protein, open these channels for a prolonged period, resulting in prolonged muscle action and the symptoms described above. This is not desirable for performance horses.

As horses with a single copy of the allele are affected, *HYPP* is dominant. Horses with two copies of the allele (homozygotes) are affected more severely. The condition can be aggravated by exercise and can be reduced by feeding a diet low in potassium. Horses with this condition all appear to be descended from a single stallion, IMPRESSIVE (1968–1995) (Bowling *et al.*, 1996). A DNA-based test has been developed, and the allele with the mutation has been designated "*H*", with the normal allele designated "*N*". The American Quarter Horse Association (AQHA) requires testing for horses descended from IMPRESSIVE, and since 2007, horses that have the genotype *H/H* are not eligible for registration. Other registries that include Quarter Horses in their ancestry have rules excluding the registration of *H/H* horses as well, or they are considering those rules. (In the case of *HYPP*, the practice of identifying genotypes using a slash to separate the alleles, i.e. *H/H*, *H/N*, *N/N*, etc., is recommended by AQHA, and is also followed by the University of California at Davis.)

The Quarter Horse breed comprises multiple populations based on use (halter, cutting, reining, racing, western pleasure, etc.), and the frequency of horses affected by HYPP ranges from 0% to 56% in the various groups (Tryon *et al.*, 2009).

Hereditary equine regional dermal asthenia (HERDA)

HERDA, formerly referred to as hyperelastosis cutis, is a hereditary disease seen primarily in Quarter Horses bred for cattle cutting. Horses appear normal at birth. Typically, the condition is found when they are first saddled. Just the pressure of the saddle and girth will cause bruising or other trauma. The skin appears to be unusually sensitive to wounds, and the wounds heal with difficulty. Affected horses are sometime euthanized owing to the severity of the condition and the associated discomfort.

Gene mapping studies led to identification of an associated chromosome region (ECA1), and based on gene function in humans, implicated a candidate gene *PPIB*, the gene for cyclophilin B (peptidylprolyl isomerase B) (Tryon *et al.*, 2007). The gene was sequenced and a mutation which substituted an amino acid in a critical folding region was subsequently shown to be completely associated with HERDA. A diagnostic DNA test exists and the trait is recessive. Carriers are unaffected. In the multiple populations of the Quarter Horse based on use (listed above under HYPP), the carrier rate for the mutation causing *HERDA* ranged from 0% to 28% (Tryon *et al.*, 2009). Two copies of the gene are necessary for the condition to occur, and as long as carriers are not mated to carriers, there will be no affected offspring.

Glycogen branching enzyme deficiency (GBED)

GBED is a condition found in Quarter Horses and related breeds. Foals may be aborted or stillborn. Those born alive appear weak and hypothermic. Affected foals die or are euthanized before 4 months of age owing to complications and the severity of the disease. Gene mapping studies localized the gene to ECA26, and a strong candidate gene in the region, the glycogen branching enzyme gene (*GBE1*), was sequenced to reveal a mutation that created a stop codon and truncated production of the enzyme (Ward *et al.*, 2004). In the absence of a functional enzyme, tissues cannot store or mobilize glycogen as a source of cellular energy. Normal parents can have affected offspring so the mutation is recessive. A diagnostic test has been developed and carriers can be identified. The carrier rate for the mutation causing *GBED* ranged from 0% to 26% in the various groups of the Quarter Horse based on use (Tryon *et al.*, 2009).

Type 1 polysaccharide storage myopathy (PSSM1)

PSSM1 is a glycogen storage disease found in draft horses, Quarter Horses, and related breeds. Clinical signs are not seen until maturity, typically around 5 years of age in Quarter Horses and 8–11 years in draft horses. Clinical signs include symptoms of muscle stiffness, sweating, reluctance to move, and weakness. A genome-wide scan implicated genes in a region of ECA10, and a strong candidate, the glycogen synthase gene (*GYS1*), was identified. Sequencing revealed a mutation in which an amino acid substitution occurred in the enzyme and this was found to be associated with PSSM1 (McCue *et al.*, 2008). The allele is dominant such that a single copy of the gene is sufficient to cause the disease.

Population studies show that the gene is rare among Shire and Morgan horses, has a prevalence of 6% to 8% in Appaloosas, Quarter Horses, and Paint horses, and a prevalence of 39% in Belgians and 62% in Percherons (McCue *et al.*, 2010). However, the severity of the disease appears to be strongly influenced by other factors, including diet, management, and breed. High glycogen diets and limited exercise heighten the effect. McCue *et al.* (2008) suggest that this mutation may have originated over 1200 years ago, and been beneficial at a time when horses may have done more work and had limited feed.

Malignant hyperthermia (MH)

MH is a well-known disease in humans, pigs, and other species. Mutations in the ryanodine receptor 1 gene (*RYR1*) in these species result in a variety of effects on muscle, but especially in an extreme sensitivity to halothane anesthesia. A mutation resulting in a substitution of an amino acid of *RYR1* was found to confer these same effects on horses (Aleman *et al.*, 2009). The condition is dominant and has a frequency of approximately 1% among Quarter Horses (McCue *et al.*, 2009). There was some evidence that the combination of the *GSY1* mutation with the *RYR1* mutation caused more severe symptoms of PSSM (McCue *et al.*, 2009). No data was available for this gene in other breeds.

Breed: Arabian horses

Severe combined immunodeficiency disease (SCID)

SCID is an uncommon disease of Arabian horses. Affected horses appear normal at birth, but their immune systems do not develop and they die of opportunistic infectious diseases within 3 months. As the disease was only seen among Arabian horses, it appeared to be hereditary. Normal parents could have affected offspring, so the disease appeared to be caused by a recessive gene. In mice, SCID occurs because of a mutation in the gene *DNA-PK*, which encodes the enzyme DNA-dependent protein kinase. Therefore, scientists considered this a candidate for the disease gene in horses, and sequenced the gene from normal and affected horses. A deletion of five DNA bases within the gene *DNA-PK* caused a frameshift mutation that prevented production of the enzyme (Shin *et al.*, 1997). The discovery of the mutation allowed the development of a diagnostic test to identify carriers of the disease gene. The occurrence of carriers among Arabian horses was found to be 8.4% in the USA (Bernoco and Bailey, 1998). Based on this rate, it was predicted that affected foals would occur at a rate of one in every 567 births. However, if breeders never mate carriers to carriers, they will never produce foals with SCID.

Lavender foal syndrome (LFS)

LFS is an uncommon disease of Arabian horses. Foals are unable to stand at birth, and exhibit multiple neurological deficiencies and a dilute coat color, referred to as lavender. The condition has been identified among Arabian horses belonging to the Egyptian Arabian lineage. Normal parents can have affected offspring, hence the disease has been regarded as a recessive trait. Similar diseases have been observed in mice and people as a result of mutations in two genes (*RAB27A* and *MYO5A*).

No families were available for LFS studies because breeders have avoided matings that produce affected horses and culled carriers. But genome-wide association studies (GWAS) of a small number of affected horses implicated the equine homologue of *MYO5A* as the most likely site of mutations causing LFS. Subsequent sequencing of the gene led to the discovery of a single base deletion in exon 30, which led to a frameshift mutation and loss of function for this gene (Brooks *et al.*, 2010). These authors developed a diagnostic test to detect carriers of LFS. They also reported a frequency of carriers among Egyptian Arabian horses of 10.3%, although they indicated that this was probably an overestimate as it was not based on a random selection of horses – only horses submitted by interested horse owners were tested. Carriers are normal and undetectable without the test, but as long as they are detected and never mated to other carriers, breeders can avoid having affected foals.

Cerebellar abiotrophy (CA)

CA occurs in Arabian horses of Polish, Egyptian, and Spanish breeding. Foals appear normal at birth, but they begin to exhibit neurological signs between 6 weeks and 4 months of age. Symptoms include ataxia, difficulty rising from a reclining position, easy to startle, a wide-based stance, and a paddling motion of the feet when moving. Family studies indicated a simple recessive trait, and carriers appeared normal. No obvious candidate genes were known.

Gene mapping and DNA sequencing led to the discovery of a SNP on ECA2 which had the potential to affect two different genes, *TOE1* and *MUTYH*, which are expressed in neural tissue (Brault *et al.*, 2011). It was not possible to determine which gene was responsible, but it was possible to develop a diagnostic test based on the DNA mutation. The authors determined that 19.2% of Arabian horses in their tests were carriers. Arabian horses have contributed to the foundation of other horse breeds, so horses of other breeds were tested for this mutation. Tests of horses from 31 other breeds only identified low frequencies of the gene in Bashkir Curly horses, Trakehners and Welsh ponies (Brault and Penedo, 2011). As stated above, the existence of a test for the recessive gene makes it possible to avoid mating carriers to carriers and producing affected offspring.

Breed: Belgian draft horses (USA)

Junctional epidermolysis bullosa (JEB-LAMC2)

JEB-LAMC2 is a tragic disease seen in newborn Belgian horse foals which causes sloughing of the skin or blistering at points of pressure. The condition causes considerable suffering to the foal and affected animals are euthanized. Defects to the laminin-5 protein cause similar diseases in other species. Laminin-5 is an integral protein for the basement membrane of cells, and three genes encode the three polypeptides that comprise the protein: *LAMA3*, *LAMB2*, and *LAMC3*. Spirito *et al.* (2002) sequenced the genes and uncovered the insertion of a nucleotide in the gene for *LAMAC2*; the insertion causes a frameshift mutation that results in the premature termination of translation. Parents of affected offspring appear normal. so a single copy of the normal gene is sufficient for normal function, i.e. the trait shows a recessive mode of inheritance. A diagnostic test has been developed, but gene frequencies and carrier rates have not been reported. Sporadic cases of JEB have been reported for draft horse breeds in Europe and may be related to this mutation. The higher frequency of JEB among American-bred Belgian draft horses is thought to be due to presence of the gene in the small foundation population initially established for these horses in the USA, and result from inbreeding. JEB also occurs in American Saddlebreds, but affected horses do not have this mutation.

Breed: American Saddlebred horses

Junctional epidermolysis bullosa (JEB-LAMA3)

JEB-LAMA3 produces pathological symptoms in American Saddlebred horses that are similar to those of JEB in Belgian horses, but has a different genetic basis. Graves *et al.* (2008) sequenced the *LAMA3* gene for affected and unaffected Saddlebreds and discovered a 6589 bp deletion spanning exons 24–27. This deletion prevents production of laminin-5 protein. Parents of affected horses are normal and the condition has a recessive mode of inheritance. A diagnostic test has been developed and 5% of a random selection of Saddlebred horses were found to be carriers. Assuming mating at random, 6.7 foals in 10,000 would be affected. Breeders can avoid the disease if they never mate affected horses to other affected horses.

Breeds: Fell and Dale ponies

Foal immunodeficiency syndrome (FIS)

FIS is tragic because foals are healthy at birth. However, their immune system does not develop and the foals succumb to opportunistic infections by the age of 3 months. The disease was initially seen among a population of Fell ponies and was called Fell pony syndrome. A hereditary basis was suspected and the mode of inheritance was thought to be recessive because the parents of affected horses were normal. The disease appeared to be similar to *SCID* in Arabian horses, but DNA tests did not uncover the same gene defect.

A genome-wide scan was conducted and genes on a region of ECA26 were implicated. The entire region of 996,000 bases was sequenced in normal and affected horses, and revealed a mutation in the sodium/myoinositol co-transporter gene (*SMIT* or *SLC5A3*) which changed a critical amino acid (Fox-Clipsham *et al.*, 2011a,b). All affected horses were homozygous for this mutation. Defects in this gene have not previously been known to cause immunodeficiency diseases in any other species. A diagnostic test was developed and horses of related breeds tested. The mutation was only found among Fell and Dale ponies, and coloured horses, with carrier rates of 38%, 18%, and 1%, respectively; no carriers were found in Clydesdales, Exmoor ponies, 161 Welsh section D, 49 part-bred Welsh section D, and 183 Highland ponies. Fell ponies are considered an endangered breed, and culling breeding stock would be disadvantageous to the genetic diversity of the breed. The test therefore makes it possible for breeders to avoid mating carriers to carriers and eliminate the possibility of having an affected offspring.

Breeds: Appaloosa, Knabstrupper, and Miniature horses

Congenital stationary night blindness (CSNB)

CSNB is a hereditary condition resulting in a loss of vision under low light conditions. The phenotype is difficult to measure and affected horses compensate for the loss of vision through behavioral modifications, including following herd mates during movement and relying on memory. CSNB appeared more prevalent among Appaloosa horses. However, the genetic basis of the condition was not clear until it was studied in connection with the gene for the appaloosa color spotting pattern (*LP*).

Gene mapping studies localized the gene for appaloosa (*LP*) to a region of ECA1 that included a candidate gene, the transient receptor potential cation channel, subfamily M, member 1 gene *(TRPM1)* (Terry *et al.*, 2004). *TRPM1* was not well characterized, though it was thought to play a role in melanin biology, and also a role in cell signaling. The expression of *TRPM1* in the skin and retina of normal and homozygous appaloosa spotted horses was found to be dramatically decreased when compared with that in other horses, demonstrating that this single gene was the most likely cause of both CSNB and the appaloosa spotting pattern (Bellone *et al.*, 2008). At the time of writing, the molecular cause of CSNB and appaloosa has not been reported; no mutations have been found within the coding regions of *TRPM1*, and it seems likely that a mutation in a regulatory region for *TRPM1* is responsible for the changes in gene expression and for CSNB (Bellone *et al.*, 2010).

Breeds: Those with white spotting patterns

Lethal white foal syndrome (LWFS)

LWFS, also called Overo Lethal White Foal Syndrome (OLWFS, or OLWS) or ileo-colonic aganglionosis, was discussed in Chapter 8, in connection with the overo color pattern manifested by horses possessing one copy of this gene. Horses with one copy of the gene have a white spotting pattern which is attractive to horse breeders. Horses with two copies of the gene have multiple developmental and neurological problems and die soon after birth. One characteristic of these foals is that they have white hair color. The condition appears similar to Hirschsprung's disease in humans, which is caused by a defect in a gene encoding the endothelin receptor type B (*EDNRB*). Therefore, scientists sequenced the equine homologue of *EDNRB* among affected and non-affected horses. Three laboratories reported the discovery of a mutation in which an amino acid substitution occurred in a critical part of the molecule (Metallinos *et al.*, 1998; Santschi *et al.*, 1998; Yang *et al.*, 1998). A diagnostic test was developed and all affected horses were found to be homozygous for the mutation. Carriers are normal with respect to the neurological disease, but do not display the overo color pattern.

Mendelian Disease Genes Not Yet Characterized at the DNA Level

As noted above, whenever a condition shows a breed or family predisposition, it may have a hereditary component. The traits described in the previous section have been characterized at the DNA level, and diagnostic tests exist to aid breeders in avoiding the production of affected offspring. The traits described below are a few of those that have been characterized as having a simple Mendelian inheritance, but neither the gene nor the mutation responsible for the disease has been yet found.

Breeds: Thoroughbreds, Standardbreds, Arabians and American Quarter Horses

Hemophilia A or Factor VIII:C deficiency

This condition is a sex-linked recessive trait reported for four breeds: Thoroughbreds, Arabians, Standardbreds, and Quarter Horses. Affected horses lack blood clotting

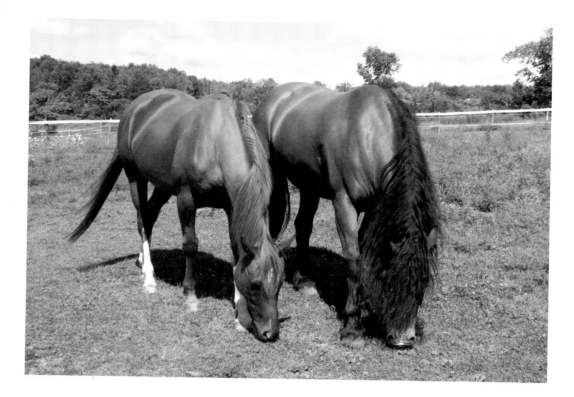

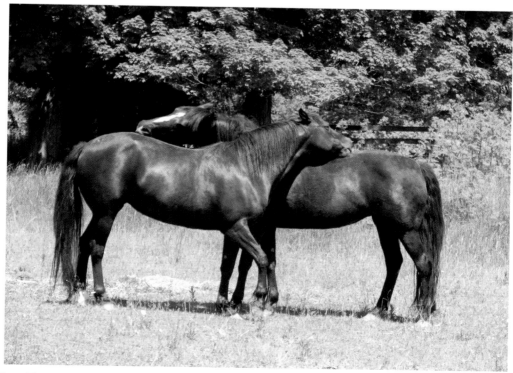

Plate 1. These Thoroughbred and draft cross mares exemplify the chestnut (left) and bay (right) base coat colors.
Plate 2. Two black Tennessee Walking horse mares.

3

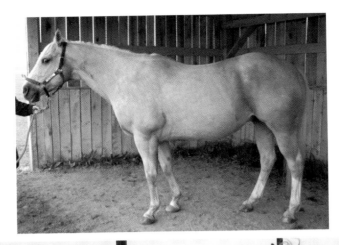

4

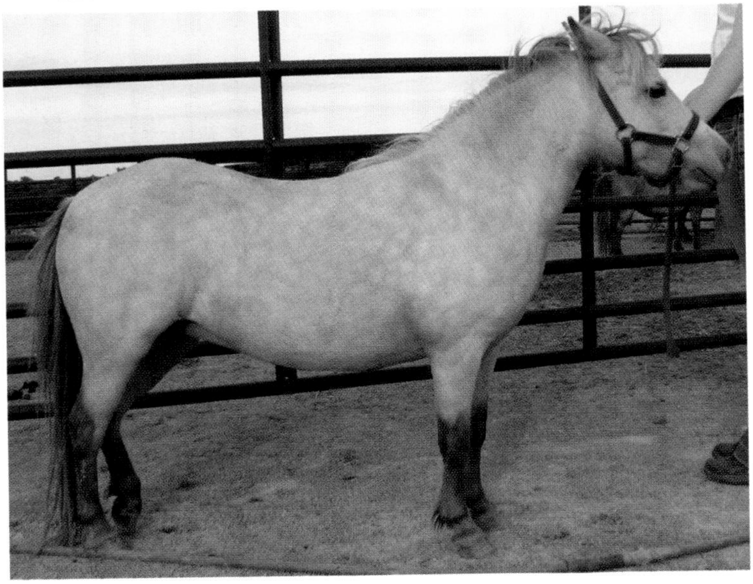

5

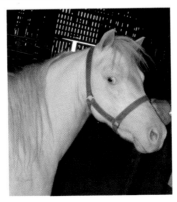

Plate 3. A palomino warmblood gelding. Palomino, a dilution of the chestnut base coat color, results in a loss of pigment from the mane and tail, and a dilution across the body.
Plate 4. This buckskin miniature horse demonstrates the darker color of the points as a result of the cream dilution on a bay base coat.
Plate 5. Blue eyes and an ivory-white coat are characteristic of horses homozygous for the *CR* allele of the *Cream Dilution* locus (*CRCR*).

6

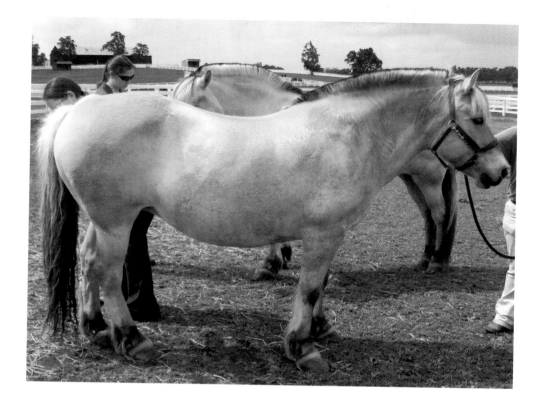

7

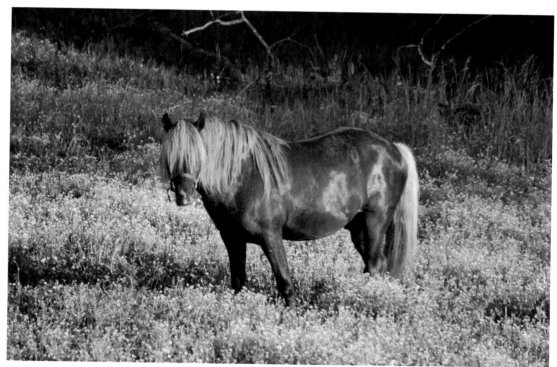

Plate 6. This dun Fjord horse possesses the unique features of this color, including a dorsal stripe and dark points.
Plate 7. Presence of the *Silver Dilution* gene has created an attractive chocolate coat color with a flaxen mane and tail on the black base coat of this Kentucky Mountain Saddle horse stallion (photo by Val Kleinheitz).

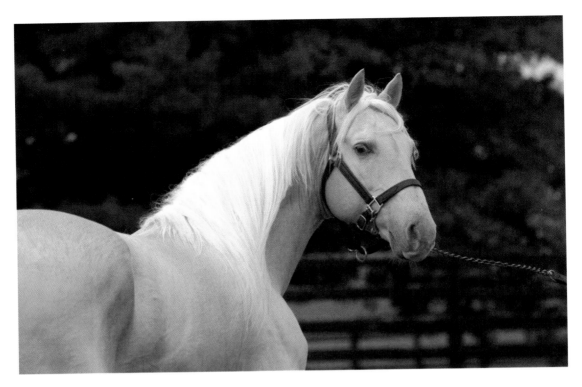

8

9

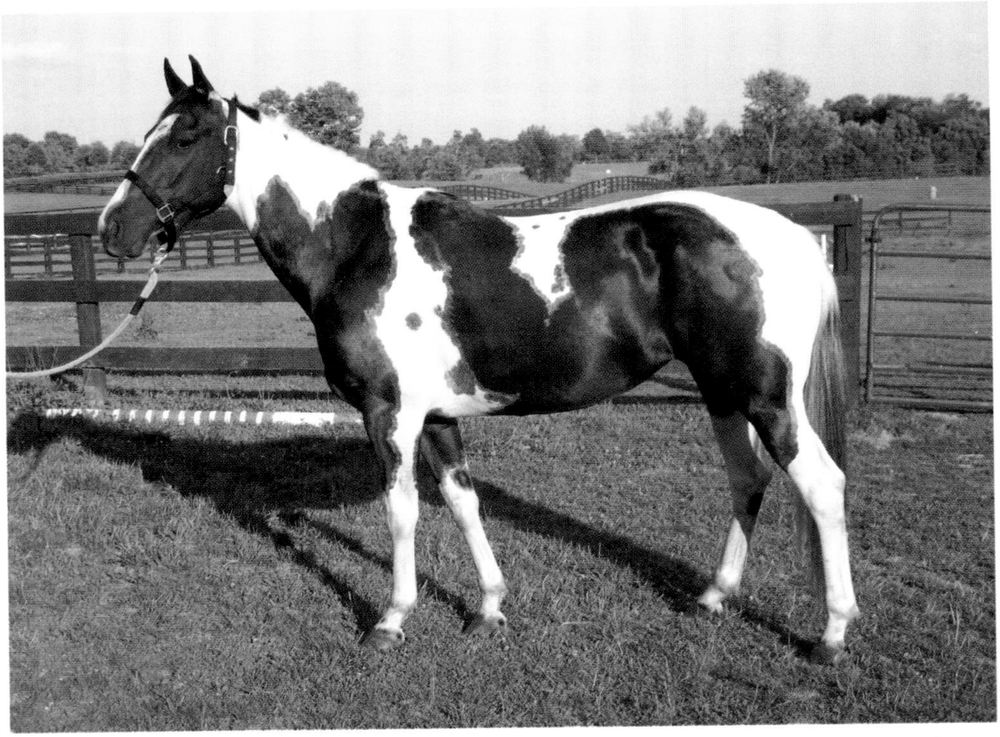

Plate 8. This gold champagne stallion displays the mottle muzzle and amber colored eye that distinguish him from a palomino (photo by Cheri Cosgrove, and kindly provided by stallion owner Val Kleinheitz).

Plate 9. The pattern of white markings known as tobiano can be associated with any basic color. This homozygous horse also possesses "ink spots", small dark patches anecdotally used to predict homozygosity.

10

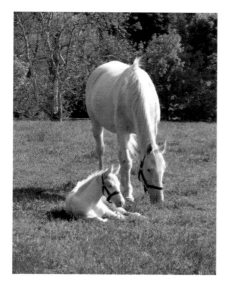

11

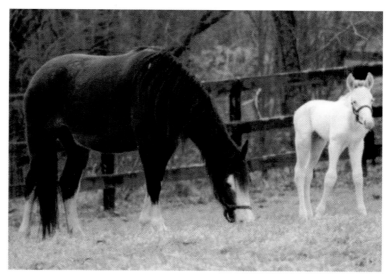

12

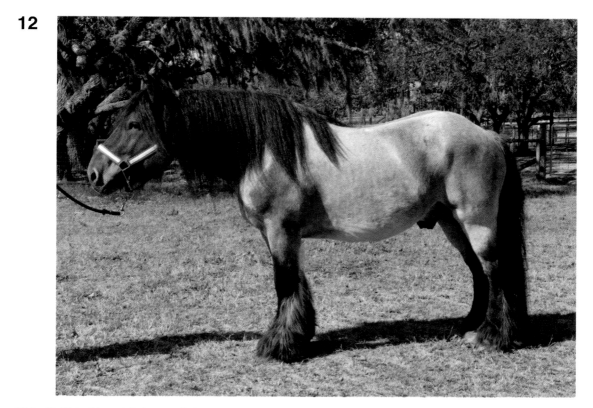

Plate 10. Pink skin and dark eyes distinguish this Thoroughbred mare and her foal as white (*Ww*), not gray (*G–*) or cremello (*Crcr*).

Plate 11. This mare and foal exemplify the pattern caused by the *Sabino1* gene. The dam is heterozygous while the foal is homozygous.

Plate 12. The interspersed mixture of light and dark hair on the body, but not the head or lower legs, characterizes the pattern produced by the *Roan* (*RN*) gene.

13

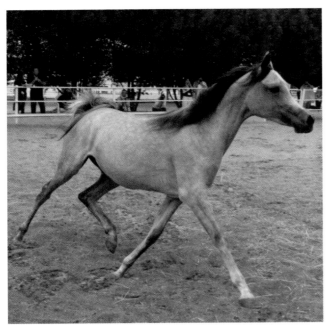

14

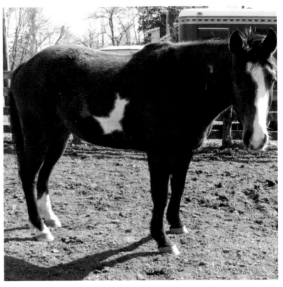

15

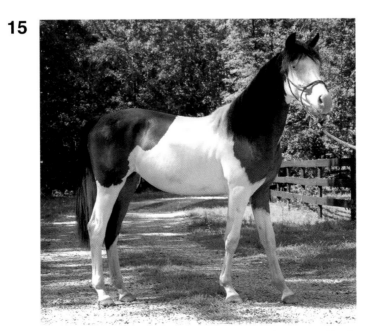

Plate 13. A yearling Arabian filly displays the typical intermediate stage of color loss caused by the *Gray* allele. Within a few years, her hair coat will be completely white, with dark skin remaining underneath.

Plate 14. Irregular white markings on the neck and sides of the barrel of this bay frame overo horse.

Plate 15. This Morgan horse mare exhibits an extensive distribution of the splashed white pattern. Her pattern is similar to that of tovero (tobiano with other white patterns), but she has been tested and is homozygous for *MITF-prom1* (*SW1*) (photo by Laura Rehning, and provided courtesy of Journey Farm Morgans).

16

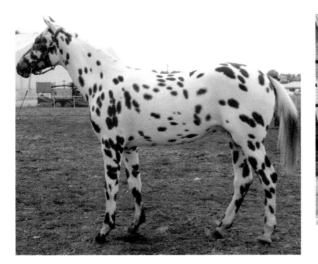

17

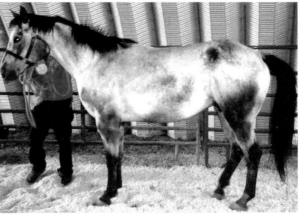

18

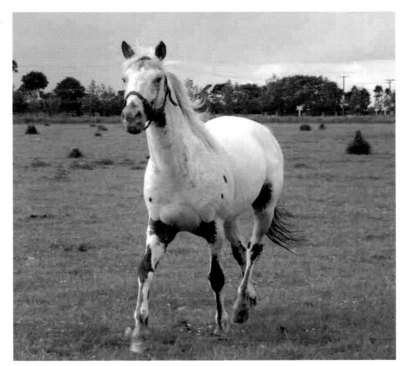

Plate 16. Horse with the leopard pattern (photo provided courtesy of Rebecca Bellone).
Plate 17. A varnished roan (or marble) leopard-patterned horse (photo provided courtesy of Rebecca Bellone).
Plate 18. A "fewspot leopard" patterned horse (photo provided courtesy of Rebecca Bellone).

19

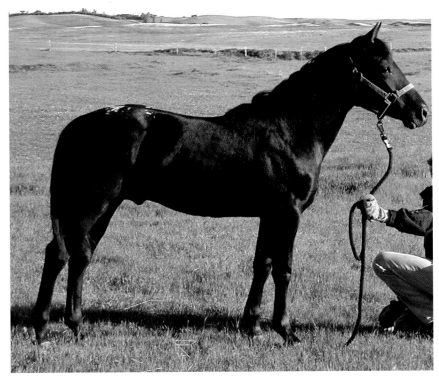

20

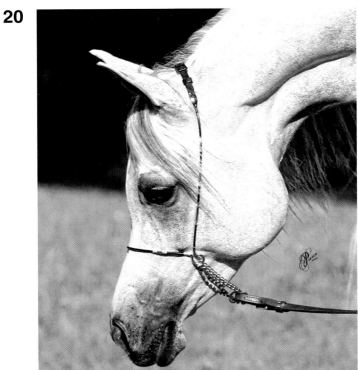

Plate 19. A leopard-patterned horse with a few white flecks on the rump (photo provided courtesy of Rebecca Bellone).
Plate 20. Gray mare exhibiting the jibbah profile that is characteristic of many Arabian horses
(photo provided courtesy of Patricia Trusty).

Factor VIII (VIII:C, the coagulant component of Factor VIII) and so they bleed excessively from wounds, or form hematomas when bruised. The gene defect has not been investigated at the DNA level, although the deficiency has been well characterized in discrete families as an X-linked recessive trait (Archer and Allen, 1972). If a horse has one normal copy of the gene for Factor VIII, then it is not affected. Because males only have one copy of the X chromosome (see Chapter 2), every time they inherit an X chromosome from the dam with the gene defect, they will be affected. Consequently, the condition is almost always seen in males. The condition is not lethal, and mature horses have been found with the defect. In the absence of molecular data, it is not apparent whether the mutations have occurred *de novo* in the different breeds or if the presence of the defect in multiple breeds reflects co-ancestry predating breed formations.

Breed: Friesian horses

Dwarfism

Dwarfism has been described in Friesian horses and results in horses with a proportionately normal head and body but shortened limbs (Fig. 12.1). Parents are normal and there appears to be a familial aspect (Back *et al.*, 2008). GWAS were conducted, and an identification made of a region harboring the gene responsible on ECA14 (Orr *et al.*, 2010). Two potential candidate genes are found in that region, but the mutation responsible for dwarfism has not yet been identified.

Breed: Miniature horses

Dwarfism

Dwarfism is also a problem for miniature horses. Breeders seek to decrease size in these horses through the accumulation of many genes, each with a modest effect on size. By contrast, a single dwarfism gene will reduce size in a single generation; however, dwarfism genes can also result in embryonic losses (Fig. 12.2) and

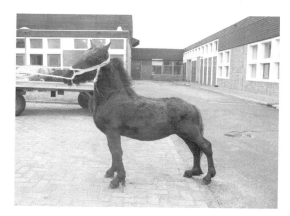

Fig. 12.1. Friesian foal with dwarfism. Notice the legs are disproportionately short compared with the back (photo provided by Dr W. Back and reprinted from Back *et al.*, 2008).

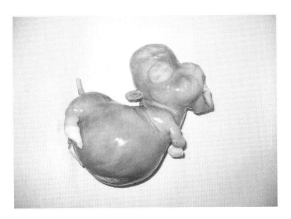

Fig. 12.2. Homozygosity for one of the dwarfism alleles resulted in this embryonic malformation resulting in abortion for an American Miniature horse (photo courtesy of John Eberth).

conformational abnormalities. GWAS have implicated a gene on ECA1 as being responsible for several different dwarfism phenotypes (Eberth and Bailey, 2010). Therefore, this is clearly not related to the dwarfism reported for Friesian horses. The specific mutations have not yet been reported, although evidence for four different mutations in the aggrecan (cartilage-specific proteoglycan core protein) gene (*ACAN*) has been presented (Eberth and Bailey, 2010). The dwarfism alleles are recessive; such that parents carrying one of the dwarfism alleles appear normal. Horses with any pair of the *ACAN* dwarfism alleles are affected, and the phenotype depends on which of the two alleles are present. Affected individuals that are heterozygous for two different *ACAN* mutations are said to be compound heterozygotes. These mutations appear to be present in miniature horses and Shetland ponies.

Breeds: Rocky Mountain, Icelandic, American Miniature, and Mountain Pleasure horses

Multiple congenital ocular anomalies (MCOA)

MCOA appear as a diverse set of ocular pathologies including abnormalities of the cornea, iris, lens, and especially, cysts in the temporal ciliary body or peripheral retina. The genetic basis of the condition was well studied in Rocky Mountain horses and found to be associated with the gene *Silver Dilution* (*SILV*). Since then, *SILV* has been found to be the result of a mutation of *PMEL17* on ECA6 (see Chapter 5). In other breeds, MCOA is not associated with *SILV* and one Rocky Mountain horse with SILV has been found with normal eyes; consequently, it is not clear which gene is responsible for MCOA (Bellone, 2010).

Complex Hereditary Diseases

Many of the diseases described above show a one-to-one correspondence between presence of the gene and presence of the disease. Diagnostic tests can be developed which are effective in identifying matings at risk of producing unhealthy offspring. But even more diseases involve the interaction, or failure of interaction, between multiple genes – or they involve an interaction between genetics and horse management. To an extent, this relationship is apparent for some of the examples described above. For instance, PSSM appears to be more severe in the presence of the gene predisposing horses to MH. Likewise, the severity of HYPP is aggravated when horses are fed diets rich in potassium.

Developmental bone diseases, arthritis, respiratory illnesses, and infectious diseases clearly involve aspects of management and environment, plus multiple organ systems – each of these with genetic influences. In the context of this book the question becomes: "To what extent does genetics influence this phenotype (disease)?" Complex traits also exhibit a range of phenotypes, extending from severely affected, to moderately affected, to unaffected. Geneticists discuss such traits as being the gene products of quantitative trait loci (QTLs), implying multiple gene effects. With this in mind, genetic studies on complex traits have two fundamental goals: (i) to identify genes with major (measurable) effects on the trait; and (ii) to measure the extent to which genetics plays a role in the trait's heritability, as determined by association in families and transmission to offspring. Below we discuss a few of the more important diseases in horses for which investigations are underway on the major genes involved and on heritability.

Examples of QTL studies

Major histocompatibility complex (MHC) associations with sarcoid tumors

The association of MHC type with diseases in horses was among the first demonstrations that genes could confer disease susceptibility. The MHC is determined by a region on ECA20 that contains genes involved in many aspects of the immune system, and is characterized by testing for lymphocyte antigens.

Lazary *et al.* (1985, 1994) summarized the results of association studies on equine leukocyte antigens with sarcoid tumors that they had conducted in families and populations of horses during the 1980s and 1990s. Sarcoid tumors are benign growths that occur in horses around the eye, in genital areas, or at sites of harness abrasions; they are induced by infections with bovine papilloma virus type 1 or type 2. Familial tendencies were observed for the occurrence of sarcoid tumors and genetic studies were conducted showing associations of MHC type in families or at the population level with the occurrence of the tumors. The association was not complete; horses could have the tumors without the MHC type or they could have the MHC type without the tumors. However, horses with the MHC lymphocyte antigen *Dw13* were 2–10 times more likely to develop sarcoid tumors than horses without the antigen, depending on breed and family. A single copy of the gene was sufficient to confer susceptibility; consequently, the susceptibility effect behaves in a dominant fashion. The variation in susceptibility between breeds and families indicated that other genes, as well as environmental factors such as exposure to the viruses, played an important role in the development of sarcoid tumors.

One value of this information was to suggest new avenues for research on this disease including discovery of interactions between the viruses and the expression of MHC genes (Marchetti *et al.*, 2009).

Osteochondrosis

Bone growth is a product of nutrition, exercise, and genetics. Osteochondrosis (OC) refers to the development of lesions in bones which may cause fragility; it may predispose horses to fracture or the creation of disassociated bone or cartilage fragments (osteochondrosis dessicans), leading to inflammation. Hereditary influences on OC have been reported by several groups using GWAS and implicating genes on ECA3 in Thoroughbred horses (Corbin *et al.*, 2011), on ECA2, ECA3, ECA13, and ECA14 in French Trotters (Teyssèdre *et al.*, 2011), on ECA5, ECA10, ECA27, and ECA28 in Norwegian Standardbreds (Lykkjen *et al.*, 2010), and on ECA2 in Hanoverian horses (Dierks *et al.*, 2010).

The diversity of these results may be perplexing, but there are two simple explanations. Firstly, the evaluation is complex, involving investigations of forelimbs, hind limbs, different radiographs, and a range of criteria and scoring systems that defy simple standardization between programs. Second, the genetic makeup of horse breeds differs, and a different constellation of genes may play a role in one breed than in another. While this makes it difficult to extrapolate the results from one study to another, the overall effect will be to provide a better understanding of all the genes that play a role in osteogenesis. Understanding the biology of bone development will provide veterinarians with a foundation for predicting the course of these diseases, and potentially lead to the discovery of therapeutic treatments to prevent or ameliorate OC in horses.

Recurrent airway obstruction (RAO)

RAO is also known as heaves or chronic hypersensitivity bronchitis is a chronic respiratory disease associated with allergy. It has long been thought to have a hereditary aspect. Marti *et al.* (1991) demonstrated a familial aspect of RAO among Swiss Warmblood and Lipizzan horses. More recently, gene mapping studies have implicated genes in regions in ECA13 for one large sire family and in ECA15 for another large sire family (Swinburne *et al.*, 2009). However, the genetic component is small compared with the role of environmental factors, including quality of hay and stabling characteristics.

Recurrent laryngeal neuropathy (RLN)

RLN was formerly referred to as idiopathic laryngeal hemiplegia. It is an obstructive upper-airway disorder caused by degeneration of the recurrent laryngeal nerves, and leading to dysfunction of the muscles served by those nerves. Affected horses will make a roaring or whistling noise during exercise, and the condition may impair performance. Heritability studies have indicated that genetics accounts for 20% of the trait in Thoroughbreds (Ibi *et al.*, 2003), and 60% in German Saddle horses (Ohnesorge *et al.*, 1993). GWAS in Thoroughbred horses have implicated regions in ECA21 and ECA31 with the *prevention* of RLN (Dupuis *et al.*, 2011).

Summary of genetic influences on disease QTLs

The diseases described in this section are only a few examples of hereditary health traits that are known or suspected for the horse. They were selected for this discussion to illustrate some of the major points regarding genetics and health. For some of these traits, environment or management is often a larger component than the genetic aspect. In effect, all horses might develop these conditions (sarcoid tumors, OC, RAO, and RLN) under the right (or wrong!) circumstances, although certain horses are more likely to succumb based on their genetic background. Understanding the basis for susceptibility to disease informs us on better management approaches for all horses. In addition, the aspects that confer susceptibility may identify targets for therapeutic or preventive treatment of all horses.

Neonatal Isoerythrolysis (NI)

NI was the first genetic disease of horses that was characterized and that led to effective health management. Also known as hemolytic disease of the newborn foal, jaundice foal disease or alloimmune hemolytic anemia of the newborn foal, the disease was initially described by Bruner *et al.* (1948). The cause of the disease is ironic as well as tragic. Foals are normal and healthy at birth, though they do not have antibodies in their blood to fight infectious diseases. During the first 24–36 h after birth, two remarkable biological events join to resolve this problem, both connected with the colostrum – the first milk of a mare, which is rich in antibodies.

The antibodies in the colostrum reflect the antibodies present in the dam's blood. In the initial 24–36 h, after birth, the gut of the foal is permeable to large protein molecules, and may even actively transport antibodies across the gut wall into the bloodstream. After this period, the dam stops concentrating antibodies in her milk, and the foal's gut becomes impermeable to proteins and begins digesting them completely into their constituent amino acids. Obtaining the colostrum is extremely important to the future health of the foal. The irony occurs when the dam produces antibodies to the red blood cells of the foal. Those antibodies will also be concentrated in the colostrum, but instead of protecting the foal, they attack its red blood cells, destroying them. Consequently, the foal is unable to effectively transfer oxygen to its tissues (one of the main functions of red blood cells). Furthermore, the products of red cell lysis are toxic to the foal, and cause jaundice and damage to multiple organs.

The first foals of mares are rarely affected. However, during the birth of this foal, some of its red blood cells stimulate the immune system of the mare. If she mounts a vigorous immune response to these red cells, and the subsequent foal has the same blood type, then the disease may occur. The only solution is to anticipate the problem: to withhold the mare's colostrum from the foal and provide colostrum from another mare that does not have antibodies to the foal's red blood cells.

Not all blood group factors are equally important as a cause of NI. Over 30 blood group antigens have been described for the horse (reviewed in Sandberg and Cothran, 2000), but most cases of NI occur as a consequence of incompatibilities for just two of the blood group factors, Aa and Qa (Stormont, 1975; Scott *et al.*, 1978). Among Thoroughbred and Standardbred mares, 1% to 2% are sensitized to Aa or Qa, and produce antibodies that may cause NI (Bailey, 1982).

Nl is considered to be a genetic disease because the blood factors involved in the immunologic reactions are inherited, and the management of the disease in sensitized mares can benefit from genetic analysis. There are no data to suggest a familial susceptibility to sensitization. Horse owners need not assume that sires or dams of affected foals possess a transmissible liability that would ethically commend their removal from a breeding pool. Once a mare has produced a foal with NI though, it is likely that subsequent foals will also be affected. It is possible to identify the type of antibody the mare produces and breed her to stallions without that factor, but in practice this is not often realistic owing to the high frequency of occurrence of the Aa and Qa factors in most breeds.

Nl disease in mule foals

Mule breeders are keenly aware that mares bred to jacks (male donkeys) can become sensitized to the blood group factors of asses (Stormont, 1975; Traub-Dargatz *et al.*, 1995). Because of this, the monitoring of a pregnant mare's serum for antibodies against the red blood cells of the jack to which she is bred is a prudent precaution to identify mule neonates at risk of Nl.

Database of Horse Diseases: Online Mendelian Inheritance in Animals (OMIA)

The influence of genetics on disease extends well beyond the examples described in this chapter. A more complete list of hereditary influences on horse diseases in can be found in the online database OMIA (see Website section for URL). The OMIA website seeks to identify and collate academic information pertinent to inherited disorders, to other (single-locus) traits, and to genes in 188 animal species. At the time of writing, it has over 200 entries for the horse, which include the examples that have been described in this chapter.

References

Aleman, M., Nieto, J.E. and Magdesian, K.G. (2009) Malignant hyperthermia associated with ryanodine receptor 1 (C7360G) mutation in Quarter Horses. *Journal of Veterinary Internal Medicine* 23, 329–334.

Archer, R.K. and Allan, B.S. (1972) True haemophilia in horses. *Veterinary Record* 91, 655–656.

Back, W., van der Lugt, J.J., Nikkels, P.G., van den Belt, A.J., van der Kiok, J.H. and Stour, T.A. (2008) Phenotypic diagnosis of dwarfism in six Friesian horses. *Equine Veterinary Journal* 40, 282–287.

Bailey, E. (1982) Prevalence of anti-red blood cell antibodies in the serum and colostrum of mares and its relationship to neonatal isoerythrolysis. *American Journal of Veterinary Research* 43, 1917–1921.

Bellone, R.R. (2010) Pleiotropic effects of pigmentation genes in horses. *Animal Genetics* 41 (Supplement 2), 100–110.

Bellone, R.R., Brooks, S.A., Sandmeyer, L., Murphy, B.A., Forsyth, G., Archer, S., Bailey, E. and Grahn, B. (2008) Differential gene expression of *TRPM1*, the likely cause of congenital stationary night blindness (CSNB) and coat spotting pattern (*LP*) in Appaloosa horses (*Equus caballus*). *Genetics* 179, 1861–1870.

Bellone, R.R., Archer, S., Wade, C.M., Cuka-Lawson, C., Haase, B., Leeb, T., Forsyth, G., Sandmeyer, L. and Grahn, B. (2010) Association analysis of candidate SNPs in *TRPM1* with leopard complex spotting (*LP*) and congenital stationary night blindness (CSNB) in horses. *Animal Genetics* 41 (Supplement 2), 207.

Bernoco, D. and Bailey, E. (1998) Frequency of the *SCID* gene in Arabian horses in the USA. *Animal Genetics* 29, 41–42.

Bowling, A.T., Byrns, G. and Spier, S. (1996) Evidence for a single pedigree source of the hyperkalemic periodic paralysis susceptibility gene in quarter horses. *Animal Genetics* 27, 279–281.

Brault, L.S. and Penedo, M.C. (2011) The frequency of the equine cerebellar abiotrophy mutation in non-Arabian horse breeds. *Equine Veterinary Journal* 43, 727–731.

Brault, L.S., Cooper, C.A., Famula, T.R., Murray, J.D. and Penedo, M.C. (2011) Mapping of equine cerebellar abiotrophy to ECA2 and identification of a potential causative mutation affecting expression of *MUTYH*. *Genomics* 97, 121–129.

Brooks, S.A., Gabreski, N., Miller, D., Brisbin, A., Brown, H.E., Streeter, C., Mezey, J., Cook, D. and Antczak, D.F. (2010) Whole-genome SNP association in the horse: identification of a deletion in myosin Va responsible for lavender foal syndrome. *PLoS Genetics* 6(4): e1000909, doi:10.1371/journal.pgen.1000909.

Bruner, D.W., Hull, E.F. and Doll, E.R. (1948) The relation of blood factors to icterus in foals. *American Journal of Veterinary Research* 9, 237–242.

Corbin, L.J. *et al.* (2011) A genome-wide association study of osteochondritis dissecans in the Thoroughbred. *Mammalian Genome* 23, 294–303.

Dierks, C., Komm, K., Lampe, V. and Distl, O. (2010) Fine mapping of a quantitative trait locus for osteochondrosis on horse chromosome 2. *Animal Genetics* 41 (Supplement 2), 87–90.

Dupuis, M.-C., Zhang, Z., Druet, T., Denoix, J.-M., Charlier, C., Lekeux, P. and Georges, M. (2011) Results of a haplotype-based GWAS for recurrent laryngeal neuropathy in the horse. *Mammalian Genome* 9–10, 613–620.

Eberth, J. and Bailey, E. (2010) Genetics of dwarfism in Miniature Horses. In: *Proceedings of the 32nd Conference of the International Society of Animal Genetics, Monday, July 26th through Friday, July 30th, 2010, Edinburgh, Scotland.* International Society of Animal Genetics p. 128, P5034 [poster].

Fox-Clipsham, L.Y., Brown, E.E., Carter, S.D. and Swinburne, J.E. (2011a) Population screening of endangered horse breeds for the foal immunodeficiency syndrome mutation. *Veterinary Record* 169, 655.

Fox-Clipsham, L.Y., Carter, S.D., Goodhead, I., Hall, N., Knottenbelt, D.C., May, P.D., Ollier, W.E. and Swinburne, J.E. (2011b) Identification of a mutation associated with fatal foal immunodeficiency syndrome in the Fell and Dales pony. *PLoS Genetics* 7(7): e1002133, doi:10.1371/journal.pgen.1002133.

Graves, K.T., Henney, P.J. and Ennis, R.B. (2009) Partial Deletion of the *LAMA3* gene is responsible for hereditary junctional epidermolysis bullosa in the American Saddlebred horse. *Animal Genetics* 40, 35–41.

Ibi, T., Miyake, T., Hobo, S., Oki, H., Ishida, N. and Sasaki, Y. (2003) Estimation of heritability of laryngeal hemiplegia in the Thoroughbred horse by Gibbs sampling. *Journal of Equine Science* 14, 81–86.

Lazary, S., Gerber, H., Glatt, P.A. and Straub, R. (1985) Equine leucocyte antigens in sarcoid-affected horses. *Equine Veterinary Journal* 17, 283–286.

Lazary, S., Marti, E., Szalai, G., Gaillard, C. and Gerber, H. (1994) Studies on the frequency and associations of equine leucocyte antigens in sarcoid and summer dermatitis. *Animal Genetics* 25 (Supplement 1), 75–80.

Lykkjen, S., Dolvik, N.I., McCue, M.E., Rendahl, A.K., Mickelson, J.R. and Roed, K.H. (2010) Genome-wide association analysis of osteochondrosis of the tibiotarsal joint in Norwegian Standardbred trotters. *Animal Genetics* 41 (Supplement 2), 111–120.

Marchetti, B., Gault, E.A., Cortese, M.S., Yuan, Z., Ellis, S.A., Nasir, L. and Campo, M.S. (2009) Bovine papillomavirus type 1 oncoprotein E5 inhibits equine MHC class I and interacts with equine MHC I heavy chain. *Journal of General Virology* 90, 2865–2870.

Marti, E., Gerber, H., Essich, G., Oulehla, J. and Lazary, S. (1991) The genetic basis of equine allergic diseases. 1. Chronic hypersensitivity bronchitis. *Equine Veterinary Journal* 23, 457–460.

McCue, M.E., Valberg, S.J., Miller, M.B., Wade, C., Akman, O., DiMauro, S. and Mickelson, J.R. (2008) Glycogen synthase (*GYS1*) mutation causes a novel skeletal muscle glycogenosis. *Genomics* 91, 458–466.

McCue, M.E., Valberg, S.J., Jackson, M., Borgia, L., Lucio, M. and Mickelson, J.R. (2009) Polysaccharide storage myopathy phenotype in Quarter Horse-related breeds is modified by the presence of an *RYR1* mutation. *Neuromuscular Disorders* 19, 37–43.

McCue, M.E., Anderson, S.M., Valberg, S.J., Piercy, R.J., Barakzai, S.Z., Binns, M.M., Distl, O., Penedo, M.C., Wagner, M.L. and Mickelson, J.R. (2010) Estimated prevalence of the type 1 polysaccharide storage myopathy mutation in selected North American and European breeds. *Animal Genetics* 41 (Supplement 2), 145–149.

Metallinos, D.L., Bowling, A.T. and Rine, J. (1998) A missense mutation in the endothelin-B receptor gene is associated with lethal white foal syndrome: an equine version of Hirschsprung disease. *Mammalian Genome* 9, 426–431.

Ohnesorge, B., Deegen, E., Miesner, K. and Geldermann, H. (1993) [Laryngeal hemiplegia in warmblood horses – a study of stallions, mares and their offspring.] *Zentralblatt für Veterinarmedizin A* 40, 134–154 [in German with English abstract].

Orr, N., Back, W., Gu, J., Leegwater, P., Govindarajan, P., Conroy, J., Ducro, B., Van Arendonk, J.A., MacHugh, D.E., Ennis, S., Hill, E.W. and Brama, P.A. (2010) Genome-wide SNP association-based localization of a dwarfism gene in Friesian dwarf horses. *Animal Genetics* 41 (Supplement 2), 2–7.

Rudolph, J., Spier, S., Byrns, G., Rojas, C., Bernoco, D. and Hoffman, E. (1992) Periodic paralysis in Quarter Horses, a sodium channel mutation disseminated by selective breeding. *Nature Genetics* 2, 144–147.

Sandberg, K. and Cothran, E.G. (2000) Biochemical genetics and blood groups. In: Bowling, A.T. and Ruvinsky, A. (eds) *The Genetics of the Horse*. CAB International, Wallingford, UK, pp. 85–108.

Santschi, E.M., Purdy, A.K., Valberg, S.J., Vrotsos, P.D., Kaese, H. and Mickelson, J.R. (1998) Endothelin receptor B polymorphism associated with lethal white foal syndrome in horses. *Mammalian Genome* 9, 306–309.

Scott, A.M. (1978) Immunogenetic analysis as a means of identification in horses. In: Bryans, J.T. and Gerber, H. (eds) *Proceedings of the Fourth International Conference on Equine Infectious Diseases*. Veterinary Publications, New Jersey, pp. 259–268.

Shin, E.K., Perryman, L.E. and Meek, K. (1997) A kinase negative mutation of *DNA-PK(CS)* in equine SCID results in defective coding and signal joint formation. *Journal of Immunology* 158, 3565–3569.

Spirito, F., Charlesworth, A., Linder, K., Ortonne, J.P., Baird, J. and Meneguzzi, G. (2002) Animal models for skin blistering conditions: absence of laminin 5 causes hereditary junctional mechanobullous disease in the Belgian horse. *Journal of Investigative Dermatology* 119, 684–691.

Stormont, C. (1975) Neonatal isoerythrolysis in domestic animals: a comparative review. *Advances in Veterinary Science and Comparative Medicine* 19, 23–45.

Swinburne, J.E., Bogle, H., Klukowska-Rötzler, J., Drögemüller, M., Leeb, T., Temperton, E., Dolf, G. and Gerber, V. (2009) A whole-genome scan for recurrent airway obstruction in

Warmblood sport horses indicates two positional candidate regions. *Mammalian Genome* 20, 504–515.

Terry, R.B., Archer, S., Brooks, S., Bernoco, D. and Bailey, E. (2004) Assignment of the Appaloosa coat colour gene (*LP*) to equine chromosome 1. *Animal Genetics* 35, 134–137.

Teyssèdre, S., Dupuis, M.C., Guérin, G., Schibler, L., Denoix, J.M., Elsen, J.M. and Ricard, A. (2012) Genome-wide association studies for osteochondrosis in French Trotter horses. *Journal of Animal Science* 90, 45–53.

Traub-Dargatz, J.L., McClure, J.J., Koch, C. and Schlipf, J.W. (1995) Neonatal isoerythrolysis in mule foals. *Journal of the American Veterinary Medical Association* 206, 67–70.

Tryon, R.C., White, S.D. and Bannasch, D.L. (2007) Homozygosity mapping approach identifies a missense mutation in equine cyclophilin B (*PPIB*) associated with HERDA in the American Quarter Horse. *Genomics* 90, 93–102.

Tryon, R.C., Penedo, M.C., McCue, M.E., Valberg, S.J., Mickelson, J.R., Famula, T.R., Wagner, M.L., Jackson, M., Hamilton, M.J., Nooteboom, S. and Bannasch, D.L. (2009) Evaluation of allele frequencies of inherited disease genes in subgroups of American Quarter Horses. *Journal of the American Veterinary Medical Association* 234, 120–125.

Ward, T.L., Valberg, S.J., Adelson, D.L., Abbey, C.A., Binns, M.M. and Mickelson, J.R. (2004) Glycogen branching enzyme (*GBE1*) mutation causing equine glycogen storage disease IV. *Mammalian Genome* 15, 570–577.

Yang, G.C., Croaker, D., Zhang, A.L., Manglick, P., Cartmill, T. and Cass, D. (1998) A dinucleotide mutation in the endothelin-B receptor gene is associated with lethal while foal syndrome (LWFS) a horse variant of Hirschsprung disease. *Human Molecular Genetics* 7, 1047–1052.

Website

Online Mendelian Inheritance in Animals, University of Sydney, New South Wales, Australia. Available at: http://omia.angis.org.au/home (accessed 10 December 2012).

13 The Horse Karyotype and Chromosomal Abnormalities

Cytogeneticists take a global view of genetics. While other geneticists study individual traits in families or sequence fragments of DNA, cytogeneticists evaluate the entire genome using the complete set of chromosomes. These scientists culture cells, count, and characterize the morphology of chromosomes. Indeed, chromosome number and morphology is characteristic of a species. Horses have 64 chromosomes, humans 46, cows 60, domestic cats 38, domestic dogs 78, etc. Chromosome numbers even vary among the different species in the genus *Equus*, as described in Chapter 18. The first accurate report for the number of horse chromosomes was by Rothfels *et al.* (1959). Since then cytogenetics has become a key tool for understanding health in horses.

Sex Chromosomes and Autosomes

Of the 64 chromosomes found in each cell of a normal, healthy horse, 32 come from the sire and 32 from the dam. Each parent contributes one sex chromosome and 31 autosomes. As noted in Chapter 2, females have two copies of the X chromosome, while males have one X and one Y chromosome. The other 31 chromosomes are referred to as autosomes to distinguish them from the sex chromosomes. The normal karyotype of a mare is designated "64,XX" denoting that she has 64 chromosomes, including two of the X sex chromosomes. Conversely, normal stallion karyotypes are designated "64,XY" denoting 64 chromosomes, including one X and one Y sex chromosome.

It is very important that horses have no less and no more than two copies of each autosome. While some minor variation may be tolerated in the structure of chromosomes, the gain, loss, or rearrangement of chromosomes is often associated with infertility, abortion, or disease. As noted below, variation in the sex chromosomes is better tolerated, although this variation is usually associated with infertility.

Cytogeneticists are scientists who can identify and evaluate abnormalities of chromosomes. This chapter describes their approaches and some of their findings.

The standard horse karyotype

The visual representation of chromosomes is called a karyotype. Karyotypes are based on a visual inspection of the number and morphology of metaphase chromosomes (which are tightly coiled during cell division) under a light microscope. The appearance of metaphase chromosomes in the microscope field is shown in Fig. 13.1. A standard karyotype for the horse was last described by a committee of equine

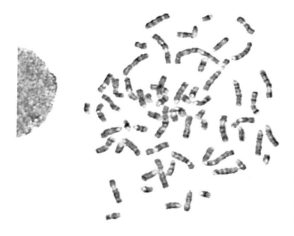

Fig. 13.1. G-banded, metaphase horse chromosomes observed with a light microscope. Notice the part of a condensed nucleus on the left of the image. (Image: T.L. Lear)

cytogeneticists in 1997 (Bowling *et al.*, 1997). The creation of an internationally accepted standard is important so that scientists will agree on the names used for chromosomes in clinical reports or in scientific studies.

The fundamental characteristics of a karyotype are:

1. The number of chromosomes.
2. The relative length of each chromosome.
3. The position of the centromere on each chromosome: the centromere is a structure which functions to accurately move chromosomes during cell division, and each normal chromosome has just one centromere.
4. The banding characteristics observed under a light microscope following treatments and staining of chromosome associated proteins. Banding methods include G-banding (treatment with trypsin and staining with Giemsa), C-banding (barium hydroxide treatment and Giemsa staining), R-banding (treatment with BrdU (5-bromo-2'-deoxyuridine), Giemsa staining, and silver staining). Each method highlights a different feature of the karyotype, but typically only one is used in routine karyotypic analysis.

Compare the chromosome images in Fig. 13.1 with those in Fig. 2.1. In Fig. 13.1, the chromosomes have been treated to exhibit G-banding.

Identifying chromosomes with fluorescence *in situ* hybridization (FISH)

More recently, scientists have used molecular techniques to track specific DNA molecules on chromosomes with a technique called fluorescence *in situ* hybridization, commonly referred to as FISH. Basically, scientists take advantage of the propensity of DNA to bind (hybridize) to DNA strands with homologous DNA sequences. DNA fragments containing specific genes are tagged with fluorescent dyes and then hybridized to chromosomes; chromosomes containing homologous genes will show fluorescence in the homologous region of the gene. In this way, chromosomes can be identified based on the specific DNA content as well as on the basis of length, configuration, and banding patterns. This approach has also been used to compare the organization of chromosomes and genes among diverse species.

Identification of chromosomes in a karyotype

A normal karyotype for a male horse is shown in Fig. 13.2. The chromosomes in this image have been treated with enzymes and stained using G-banding. The bands correspond to regions in which proteins are tightly bound to the DNA in regions called heterochromatin. According to tradition, chromosome 1 is the longest chromosome, and has a centromere appearing near the middle of the chromosome. Depending on the position of the centromere, this is referred to as metacentric (middle), or submetacentric (near middle). All of the metacentric and submetacentric chromosomes are numbered from largest to smallest. Next, the chromosomes with the centromere at the end of the chromosome are numbered, again from largest to smallest. When the centromere is at the end, it is referred to as acrocentric or telocentric. The horse has 13 metacentric or submetacentric chromosomes, numbered 1–13, followed by another 18 acrocentric chromosomes numbered 13–31. The last two chromosomes are the X and Y chromosomes. The X chromosome is a large metacentric while the Y chromosome is a very small acrocentric chromosome. As noted earlier in the book, chromosomes 1–31 occur in duplicates, one inherited from the male and the other from the female. The X and Y chromosomes are profoundly different from each other in their appearance and content, except for a very small section called the pseudoautosomal region; this allows the X and Y chromosomes to behave as a normal pair of chromosomes during cell division.

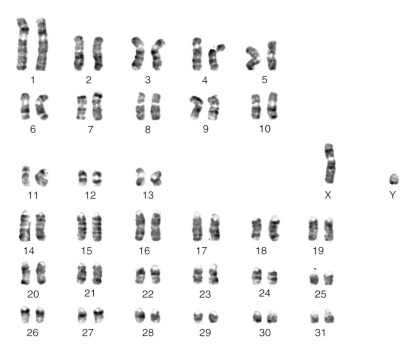

Fig. 13.2. Images of horse chromosomes have been captured and arrayed to show the 32 characteristic pairs found in the horse. This G-banded karyotype shows the 31 autosomes plus the X and Y chromosomes found in a male horse. (Image: T.L. Lear)

Chapter 13

Another convention of cytogenetics is to include a species designation along with the numbering of a chromosome. The species designation is based on the first letter of the genus (*Equus*) and the first two letters of the species (*caballus*). Therefore, horse chromosome 1 is designated ECA1. Likewise, the largest chromosome for donkeys (*Equus asinus*) is designated EAS1 and the largest chromosome for people (*Homo sapiens*) is designated HSA1.

As well as the length and morphology of the chromosomes, cytogeneticists use banding patterns to precisely identify them. When using the international agreement for nomenclature, we can be confident that scientists in Sweden, the USA, Japan, and Australia will accurately refer to the same chromosome in their clinical and scientific reports.

Variation in Chromosome Arrangements

Mosaicism

Sometimes all the cells in a karyotype analysis do not have the same number or configuration of autosomes. This may occur when an error occurs during early cell division in the embryo, and a chromosome is lost or damaged. If the cell remains viable, despite the damage, all cells descended from that cell will exhibit the same karyotypic characters. Mosaic is the term used to describe the situation where some cells in a tissue exhibit the original karyotype and others exhibit the mutation.

Typically, cytogeneticists evaluate 100 or more cells to detect the occurrence of chromosome mosaicism in the individual. Alteration of a chromosome associated with loss or gain of genes for the cell is often lethal for that cell, and may result in embryonic lethal events, although if the chromosome alterations are not too great and the percentage of normal cells is sufficient, then the embryo may survive. Chromosome variation is often found to be associated with mosaicism of normal and abnormal cells. For example, a mare with both normal cells (64,XX) and cells lacking an X chromosome (63,X) would be identified as having a karyotype 63,X/64,XX. The phenotype is then characteristic of the ratio of normal and abnormal cells in the tissue.

Chromosome polymorphisms not associated with disease

The primary reason to karyotype a horse is to investigate the possibility of disease detected being a chromosome abnormality. The approach is to create a karyotype for the horse in question then compare the result with the standard karyotype for normal healthy horses. The presence of any variation between the two may be evidence of a chromosome abnormality responsible for the disease. However, some variation can occur among karyotypes without being associated with disease. Variation has been seen among healthy horses in the size of a heterochromatin block on ECA13 (Buckland *et al.*, 1976; Ryder *et al.*, 1978), presence of a structure called a nucleolus organizer region (NOR) (Kopp *et al.*, 1988), and size of the Y chromosome (Power, 1988). Other variants have been observed among horses for banding (primary heterochromatin), and in the presence of terminal structures and conformation that have not been formally reported but are known to cytogeneticists (Lear, personal communication). Therefore, simply identifying variation between horses does not necessarily constitute evidence that the variant is responsible for the disease or infertility.

Diseases associated with gain or loss of autosomes

Animals are very sensitive to disruptions in the number of chromosomes. Normal, healthy horses have two copies of all genes on autosomes, one inherited from the dam and one from the sire. Occasionally, an error may occur during meiosis that results in an egg or sperm with an extra chromosome.

When there are three copies of a particular chromosome in an embryo, the situation is called trisomy for that chromosome. Among people, Down's syndrome is the situation in which trisomy occurs for HSA21. Trisomy appears to be rare among horses, and only eight cases have been reported in the scientific literature (summarized in Lear and Villagómez, 2011). Foals with multiple developmental defects were discovered to have trisomy of ECA23 (Klunder et al., 1989), ECA26 (Bowling and Millon, 1990), ECA27 (Buoen et al., 1997), and ECA28 (Power, 1987); there were two cases each for ECA30 (Bowling and Millon, 1990; Kubień and Tischner, 2002) and ECA31 (Lear et al., 1999; Lear and Villagómez, 2011). These trisomies all involved the smallest horse chromosomes; it is likely that trisomy for the larger chromosomes entails too much genetic imbalance and results in embryonic death. Many trisomic foals that do reach term die shortly after birth or are euthanized as a consequence of their severe deformities.

While the karyotype of a normal stallion or mare is represented as 64,XY or 64,XX, cytogeneticists report a colt with trisomy for ECA 31 as "65,XY,+31" indicating a total of 65 chromosomes, and the presence of an X and Y chromosome and an additional copy of ECA31.

No examples have been found in which there has been a complete loss of an autosome in a horse, or the presence of more than three copies of an autosome, though there are reports of fragments of chromosomes being lost or present in triplicate (Durkin et al., 2011; Lear and Villagómez, 2011). The deletion or gain of these chromosome fragments came to the attention of veterinarians because of health or fertility problems.

Fertility problems associated with autosome rearrangements

Chromosomes are very stable, although a piece may occasionally break off and become attached to another chromosome. When rearrangement occurs without the loss of DNA, it is called a balanced chromosome translocation. Horses with balanced translocations have two copies of all genes and, unless the breakage has destroyed the normal function of some of the genes, they appear as normal healthy horses. The condition is rare, and only five cases have been reported among mares (Power, 1991; Lear and Layton, 2002; Lear et al., 2008; Lear and Villagómez, 2011) and two among stallions (Long, 1996; Durkin et al., 2011). While horses with balanced translocations of chromosomes appear normal in most respects, including athletic abilities, they usually experience a decrease in fertility. The problem has to do with the behavior of chromosomes during the creation of sperm and eggs (meiosis).

During meiosis, chromosomes pair and exchange material; then one centromere from each pair is pulled by microtubules to opposite poles of the cells, followed by cell division. The result is two new cells, each with only one copy of each chromosome. As each sperm and egg have only one copy of each chromosome, the union of gametes during fertilization results in an embryo with two copies of every chromosome, one inherited from the sire and one inherited from the dam.

However, when parts of one chromosome are translocated to another, it is possible to produce sperm or eggs with unbalanced genetic material. As shown in Fig. 13.3, a horse with a balanced translocation involving ECA1 and ECA16 would produce six types of gametes: one normal, one with a balanced translocation, and at least four that are defective, containing unbalanced amounts of genetic material). Embryos produced with unbalanced gametes are usually lost early in pregnancy. Horses with balanced translocations may be able to produce viable offspring, but they are less fertile because half of their gametes will be defective. Mares may become pregnant but lose embryos before day 65 of gestation. This condition in mares is referred to as repeated early embryonic loss (REEL) (Lear *et al.*, 2008).

Gain or loss of sex chromosomes

Loss of the X chromosome

The most common chromosome abnormality is the loss of the X or Y chromosome (Power, 1990). During meiosis, sperm or eggs may be created without an X or Y chromosome. If that egg or sperm joins with its counterpart possessing a single X chromosome, the result is a female with the karyotype 63,X, specifically missing

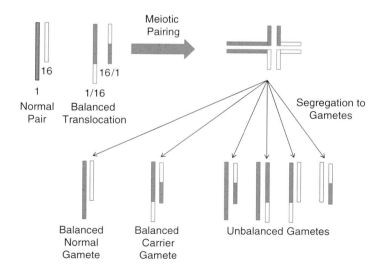

Fig. 13.3. This cartoon illustrates the potential consequences of having balanced chromosome translocations during meiosis. Sometimes the gamete receives a full complement of genes and sometimes it receives an unbalanced set. Fertilization with unbalanced gametes usually results in failure of development beyond the embryonic stage.

an X chromosome. Mares with this chromosome abnormality have small, inactive ovaries, and abnormal or absent estrus cycles; they are rarely fertile. Affected mares are commonly referred to as "XO mares" and, while viable, sometimes exhibit angular limb deformities, small stature, and poor conformation. Chromosomal mosaicism involving the loss of an X chromosome is a common finding among such mares (63,X/64,XX) (Power, 1990). Several cases have also been reported in which infertile mares were found with deletions on one of their X chromosomes, and these appeared to exhibit characteristics typical of XO mares (Bowling *et al.*, 1987).

Among people, the loss of the X chromosome is also the most common chromosome abnormality and is called Turner syndrome. Turner syndrome in women results in more severe clinical signs than the XO condition of mares, probably because of differences in the genes found on their respective X chromosomes.

Gain of X chromosomes

Three cases have been reported of mares with trisomy X (65,XXX) (Chandley *et al.*, 1975; Bowling *et al.*, 1987). While women with X trisomy are fertile, these mares had normal external genitalia, but poorly developed ovaries and infertility.

Several cases have been reported of males with extra X chromosomes, e.g. 65,XXY and 66,XXXY (Gluhovschi *et al.*, 1970; Kubień *et al.*, 1993; Mäkinen *et al.*, 2000). In these cases, the presence of the Y chromosome was sufficient for the horse to develop the stallion phenotype, but it was infertile. Among men, the 47,XXY karyotype is called Kleinfelter syndrome and is also associated with infertility.

Gain of Y chromosomes

So far, no cases have been found in which horses possess the karyotype 65,XYY or any other combination with multiple copies of the Y chromosome. However, two reports have been published for individuals with mosaic karyotypes 63,X/65,XYY (Höhn *et al.*, 1980; Paget *et al.*, 2001). Presumably, the mosaic situation came about as a result of failure of the Y chromosome to migrate to each of the new cells during the first mitotic cell divisions, resulting in a population of 63,X cells and a population of 65,XYY cells. The resulting horses exhibited intersex phenotypes: specifically, individuals with external genitalia bearing both male and female characteristics.

Disorders of Sexual Development (DSD)

At the beginning of embryonic development, the gonads are equally capable of becoming female (ovaries) or male (testis). The eventual sex of the individual is determined by which sex chromosomes are present. When a normal Y chromosome is present, the gonads become testes. In the absence of a Y chromosome, the gonads become ovaries. Abnormal numbers of the sex chromosomes can result in undeveloped genitalia, genitalia possessing characteristics of both males and females, two sets of genitalia (including ovaries and testes) or individuals possessing genitalia inconsistent with their genetic constitution, e.g. males with a female karyotype (64,XX) and females with a male karyotype (64,XY). Collectively, these conditions are referred to as disorders of sexual development, or DSD.

The most readily detected cause of DSD in horses is mosaicism in which both male and female cells are present. Several cases have been reported of individuals possessing the mosaic karyotype 63,X/64,XY (Villagómez *et al.*, 2011; reviewed in Lear and McGee, 2012). The extent of DSD depends on the proportion of cells of each type that is present in the gonadal tissue.

Often, the cause of DSD is subtle and not detectable by karyotypic analysis. Detection relies on the application of molecular genetics, based on the fact that each of the X and Y chromosomes contains unique genes that are important for development. While the X chromosome has been estimated to contain 579 protein coding genes (ENSEMBL project, see Chapter 3), the Y chromosome is much smaller – so far, only 37 genes have been identified on this chromosome (Paria *et al.*, 2011), although there are likely to be twice as many based on comparison with the human Y chromosome (86 genes). Each chromosome contains unique genes that are important for development.

XY sex reversal

One of the most common causes of DSD involves defects of the *SRY* gene, the sex determining region of the Y chromosome. *SRY* initiates a cascade of expression by other genes resulting in the development of male characteristics. When mutations simply delete the *SRY* gene from the Y chromosome, the individual will have a 64,XY karyotype typical of a male, but a female phenotype. This is sometimes called an XY "sex reversal", and it is one of the most common types of DSD. A hypothesis has been advanced that the molecular structure of this region of the Y chromosome predisposes this gene to mutation during meiosis (Raudsepp *et al.*, 2010). Defects in other genes, including *SOX-9*, which encodes the transcription factor SOX-9, and is responsible for testis development, may also result in DSD. This is an active area of research.

Some cases of DSD are not due to sex chromosome defects. A family of Arabian horses has been reported in which the occurrence of XY sex reversal was hereditary but appeared to be the product of an autosomal gene (Kent *et al.*, 1986). The genetic basis for this condition has not been determined. It may be the consequence of an androgen receptor defect encoded by an autosomal gene.

XX sex reversal

Three cases have been reported in which horses with a 64,XX karyotype had ambiguous genitalia or developed ovotestes (Vaughan *et al.*, 2001; Bannasch *et al.*, 2007; Villagómez *et al.*, 2008). All three horses were tested and found to be negative for the *SRY* gene, suggesting that the molecular defect lay elsewhere.

Prevalence of Chromosome Abnormalities Among Horses

Karyotyping is not a routine activity for horses. Only when a horse is born with developmental abnormalities, has intersex characteristics, or is found to be infertile, is karyotyping used to investigate the problem. We do not know the rate at which chromosome abnormalities occur in the random population of horses. To determine the prevalence of chromosome abnormalities, Bugno *et al.* (2007) evaluated the cytogenetics of 500 randomly selected horses of diverse breeds. Among these 500 horses, they found ten mares (2.0%) with chromosome abnormalities, nine involving sex chromosome abnormalities and one with a mosaicism for autosomal trisomy (64,XX/65,XX +31). The trisomic horse was an 11 month old mare that appeared to be phenotypically normal; only 6.8% of her cells were trisomic.

Another study used a molecular pre-screening test to detect chromosome abnormalities. Kakoi *et al.* (2005) used a microsatellite marker (LEX003) from the X chromosome to detect potential sex chromosome anomalies among 17,421 newborn foals. Suspected anomalies were further tested with karyotyping or molecular tests for additional genetic markers found on the X and Y chromosomes. These authors uncovered 18 cases of sex chromosome abnormalities, corresponding to 0.1% of the population. Considering the screening method, this is clearly an underestimate, but it indicted a potential for using molecular marker testing to identify putative chromosome abnormalities among foals.

Genomics and Cytogenetics

Molecular genetics technologies have made it possible to detect chromosomal rearrangements that occur at levels undetectable by microscopy. In fact, duplication or loss of small regions of chromosome appear to be common in all species. These types of genetic variants are called copy number variants (CNVs). Thousands of CNVs have been reported for the horse in studies comparing 16 horses from 15 breeds (Doan *et al.*, 2012). The question becomes: at what level does the gain or loss of DNA have an impact on health and fertility of a horse? Two issues are involved: (i) the presence or absence of particular genes essential to health; and (ii) the proper segregation of chromosomes during meiosis and mitosis.

Microscopic evaluation of chromosomes is usually sufficient to detect major chromosomal rearrangements. However, cytogeneticists occasionally investigate cases in which the phenotype appears to be characteristic of a chromosome abnormality but this is not apparent by microscopy. In these cases, the phenotype may be a consequence of chromosomal rearrangement or CNVs that fall below the resolution of microscopy. At present, several approaches are being developed to investigate chromosomal rearrangements using genomic tools that include SNP evaluations (see Chapters 3 and 11) and array comparative genome hybridization (array CGH). These approaches will become useful tools for clinical cytogenetics in the future (Lear and Bailey, 2008).

References

Bannasch, D., Rinaldo, C., Millon, L., Latson, K., Spangler, T., Hubberty, S., Galuppo, L. and Lowenstine, L. (2007) SRY negative 64,XX intersex phenotype in an American Saddlebred horse. *Veterinary Journal* 173, 437–439.
Bowling, A.T. and Millon, L.V. (1990) Two autosomal trisomies in the horse: 64,XX,-26,+t (26q26q) and 65,XX,+30. *Genome* 33, 679–682.

Bowling, A.T., Millon, L. and Hughes, J.P. (1987) An update of chromosomal abnormalities in mares. *Journal of Reproduction and Fertility. Supplement* 35, 149–155.

Bowling, A.T., Breen, M., Chowdhary, B.P., Hirota, K., Lear, T., Millon, L.V., Ponce de Leon, F.A., Raudsepp, T. and Stranzinger, G. (Committee) (1997) International system for cytogenetic nomenclature of the domestic horse: Report of the Third International Committee for the Standardization of the Domestic Horse Karyotype, Davis, CA, USA, 1996. *Chromosome Research* 5, 433–443.

Buckland, R.A., Fletcher, J.M. and Chandley, C. (1976) Characterization of the domestic horse (*Equus caballus*) karyotype using G- and C-banding techniques. *Experientia* 32, 1146–1149.

Bugno, M., Słota, E. and Kościelny, M. (2007) Karyotype evaluation among young horse populations in Poland. *Schweizer Archiv für Tierheilkunde* 149, 227–232.

Buoen, L.C., Zhang, T.Q., Weber, A.F., Turner, T., Bellamy, J. and Ruth, G.R. (1997) Arthrogryposis in the foal and its possible relation to autosomal trisomy. *Equine Veterinary Journal* 29, 60–62.

Chandley, A.C., Fletcher, J., Rossdale, P.D., Peace, C.K., Ricketts, S.W., McEnery, R.J., Thorne, J.P., Short, R.V. and Allen, W.R. (1975) Chromosome abnormalities as a cause of infertility in mares. *Journal of Reproduction and Fertility. Supplement* 23, 377–383.

Doan, R., Cohen, N., Harrington, J., Veazy, K., Juras, R., Cothran, G., McCue, M.E., Skow, L. and Dindot, S.V. (2012) Identification of copy number variants in horses. *Genome Research* 22, 899–907.

Durkin, K.W., Raudsepp, T. and Chowdhary, B.P. (2011) Cytogenetic evaluation. In: McKinnon, A.O., Squires, E.L., Vaala, W.E. and Varner, D.D. (eds) *Equine Reproduction*, 2nd edn. Wiley-Blackwell, Chichester, UK, pp. 1462–1468.

Gluhovschi, N., Bistriceanu, M., Suciu, A. and Bratu, M. (1970) A case of intersexuality in the horse with type 2A+XXXY chromosome formula. *British Veterinary Journal* 126, 522–525.

Höhn, H., Klug, E. and Rieck, G.W. (1980) A 63,XO/65,XYY mosaic in a case of questionable equine male pseudohermaphroditism. *Proceedings of the 4th European Colloquium on Cytogenetics of Domestic Animals, June 10–13, 1980, Uppsala, Sweden.* Department of Animal Breeding and Genetics, Faculty of Veterinary Medicine, Swedish University of Agricultural Sciences, Uppsala, Sweden, pp. 82–92.

Kakoi, H., Hirota, K., Gawahar, H., Kurosawa, M. and Kuwajima, M. (2005) Genetic diagnosis of sex chromosome aberrations in horses based on parentage test by microsatellite DNA and analysis of X- and Y-linked markers. *Equine Veterinary Journal* 37, 143–147.

Kent, M., Shoffner, R., Bouen, L. and Weber, A.F. (1986) XY sex reversal syndrome in the domestic horse. *Cytogenetics and Cell Genetics* 2, 8–17.

Klunder, L.R., McFeely, R.A., Beech, J. and McClune, W. (1989) Autosomal trisomy in a Standardbred colt. *Equine Veterinary Journal* 21, 69–70.

Kopp, E., Mayr, B. and Schleger, W. (1988) Ribosomal RNA expression in a mammalian hybrid, the hinny. *Chromosoma* 96, 434–436.

Kubień, E.M. and Tischner, M. (2002) Reproductive success of a mare with a mosaic karyotype: 64,XX/65,XX,+30. *Equine Veterinary Journal* 34, 99–100.

Kubień, E.M., Pozor, M.A. and Tischner, M. (1993) Clinical, cytogenetic and endocrine evaluation of a horse with a 65,XXY karyotype. *Equine Veterinary Journal* 25, 333–335.

Lear, T. and Bailey, E. (2008) Equine clinical cytogenetics: past and future. *Cytogenetics and Genome Research* 120, 42–49.

Lear, T.L. and Layton, G. (2002) Use of zoo-FISH to characterise a reciprocal translocation in a Thoroughbred mare: t(1;16)(q16;q21.3). *Equine Veterinary Journal* 34, 207–209.

Lear, T.L. and McGee, R.B. (2012) Disorders of sexual development in the domestic horse, *Equus caballus. Sexual Development* 6, 61–71.

Lear, T.L. and Villagomez, D.A.F. (2011) Cytogenetic evaluation of mares and foals. In: McKinnon, A.O., Squires, E.L., Vaala, W.E. and Varner, D.D. (eds) *Equine Reproduction*, 2nd edn. Wiley-Blackwell, Chichester, UK, pp. 1951–1962.

Lear, T.L., Cox, J.H. and Kennedy, G.A. (1999) Autosomal trisomy in a Thoroughbred colt: 65,XY,+31. *Equine Veterinary Journal* 31, 85–88.

Lear, T.L., Lundquist, J., Zent, W.W., Fishback, W.D. Jr and Clark, A. (2008) Three autosomal chromosome translocations associated with repeated early embryonic loss (REEL) in the domestic horse (*Equus caballus*). *Cytogenetic and Genome Research* 120, 117–122.

Long, S.E. (1996) Tandem 1;30 translocation: a new structural abnormality in the horse (*Equus caballus*). *Cytogenetic and Cellular Genetics* 72, 162–163.

Mäkinen, A., Katila, T., Andersson, M. and Gustavsson, I. (2000) Two sterile stallions with XXY-syndrome. *Equine Veterinary Journal* 32, 358–360.

Paget, S. *et al.* (2001) 63,XO/65,XYY mosaicism in a case of equine male pseudohermaphroditism. *Veterinary Record* 148, 24–25.

Paria, N., Raudsepp, T., Pearks Wilkerson, A.J., O'Brien, P.C., Ferguson-Smith, M.A., Love, C.C., Arnold, C., Rakestraw, P., Murphy, W.J. and Chowdhary, B.P. (2011) A gene catalogue of the euchromatic male-specific region of the horse Y chromosome: comparison with human and other mammals. *PLoS One* 6(7):e21374, doi: 10.1371/journal.pone.0021374.

Power, M.M. (1987) Equine half sibs with an unbalanced X;15 translocation or trisomy 28. *Cytogenetic and Cellular Genetics* 45, 163–168.

Power, M.M. (1988) Y chromosome length variation and its significance in the horse. *Journal of Heredity* 79, 311–313.

Power, M.M. (1990) Chromosomes of the horse. In: McFeely, R.A. (ed.) *Domestic Animal Cytogenetics. Advances in Veterinary Science and Comparative Medicine, Vol. 34.* Academic Press, San Diego, California, pp. 131–167.

Power, M.M. (1991) The first description of a balanced reciprocal translocation [t(1q;3q)] and its clinical effects in a mare. *Equine Veterinary Journal* 23, 146–149.

Raudsepp, T., Durkin, K., Lear, T.L., Das, P.J., Avila, F., Kachroo, P. and Chowdhary, B.P. (2010) Molecular heterogeneity of XY sex reversal in horses. *Animal Genetics* 41 (Supplement 2), 41–52.

Rothfels, K.H., Alexrad, A.A., Siminovitch, L. and McCulloch Parker, R.C. (1959) The origin of altered cell lines from mouse, monkey and man, as indicated by chromosome and transplantation studies. In: Begg, R.W. (ed.) *Proceedings of 3rd Canadian Cancer Research Conference, 1958.* Academic Press, New York, pp. 189–214.

Ryder, O.A., Epel, N.C. and Benirschke, K. (1978) Chromosome banding studies of the Equidae. *Cytogenetic and Cellular Genetics* 20, 332–350.

Vaughan, L., Schofield, W. and Ennis, S. (2001) *SRY*-negative XX sex reversal in a pony: a case report. *Theriogenology* 55, 1051–1057.

Villagómez, D.A.F., Lear, T.L., Chenier, T., Lee, S., Cahill, J., Reyes, E. and King, W.A. (2008) Equine XY and XX sex-reversal syndrome in SRY positive and negative mares. In: *Proceedings of the 18th International Colloquium on Animal Cytogenetics and Gene Mapping (18th ICACGM), June 8–10, 2008, Bucharest, Romania. Chromosome Research* 16, 1040 (abstract).

Villagómez, D.A., Lear, T.L., Chenier, T., Lee, S., McGee, R.B., Cahill, J., Foster, R.A., Reyes, E., St John, E. and King, W.A. (2011) Equine disorders of sexual development in 17 mares including XX, *SRY*-negative, XY, *SRY*-negative and XY, *SRY*-positive genotypes. *Sexual Development* 5, 16–25.

14 Genetics of Performance

Performance is at the crux of horsemanship. Horses pull, carry, and move with strength, efficiency, and grace. Accomplishments on the track, in the ring, or on the field are usually preceded by days, months, and even years of training to perfect different skills. Effective trainers discern innate athletic strengths and weaknesses of horses and then accommodate deficiencies through skillful management.

Nevertheless, skillful training will not make a Percheron horse competitive with a Thoroughbred racehorse on a mile track. Conversely, the Thoroughbred will not be able to keep up with a draft horse in a plowing or pulling competition. Genetic differences exist among horses and these are responsible for innate abilities to race, pull, plow, jump, and perform a wide range of gaits. Over the millennia, since horse domestication, people have selected horses for different characteristics, which has led to the creation of diverse breeds. Form and color have been important, but performance is the ultimate goal of breeders. Horse competitions occur among all cultures with the goal of celebrating superior performance and learning how to improve our livestock. Clearly, performance has a genetic component because we see vast differences among horses and breeds. Breeders recognize this and select superior performing horses for breeding stock.

There are three basic aspects of the genetics of performance:

1. Determining heritability of a trait within a breed
2. Determining the estimated breeding value for individuals
3. Discovery of the genes that influence performance traits.

Heritability of Performance Traits

Heritability describes the variation of a performance trait that is a consequence of genetics and is independent of management, luck, or training. The statistical approaches for determining heritability fall outside the scope of this book, but we ought to note here that horse breeders should have an understanding of the general nature of heritability measures. The single most important point here is that heritability is a characteristic of a population, and the specific genes that contribute to a phenotype may vary greatly in different populations.

Consider the genetics of racing performance as an example. We should not be surprised to learn that Thoroughbred horses have more genes that contribute significantly to racing than are found among Percheron horses. We do not study the heritability of speed among Percherons because: (i) speed is not the reason for owning Percherons; and (ii) genes that would contribute to speed among Percherons may be different from those found in Thoroughbreds. If we were to study the genetics of speed among draft horses, we might find that selection for decreased size or weight led to the greatest improvement in race track times. Perhaps lighter horses might run faster, but Thoroughbred horses are already lighter than most Percherons, so reduction in weight may not have an effect for Thoroughbreds. Instead, genes related to muscle physiology might be more significant for Thoroughbred racing performance than genes related to size. This is an important point: heritability is characteristic of a particular population or breed, and is related to the particular constellation of genes that they possess as a consequence of their origin and prior selection.

Heritability versus major genes

Much of this book focusses on specific genes that influence specific traits. We know the mutations responsible for many coat color patterns, several diseases, and even some performance characteristics. We call these "major genes", and can define their effects biochemically and physiologically. However, most traits cannot be explained by the effect of a single or even a few major genes. Instead, the phenotype is a product of interactions by tens or even hundreds of genes. Furthermore, most traits probably cannot be explained by the effect of a single or even a few major genes. This was recognized early in the 1900s, and so scientists developed methods to quantify the genetic contribution to variation among horses, and to represent that as the value that we call heritability.

The foundation for this approach is the "infinitesimal model" of R.A. Fisher developed in the 1930s. This is based on three fundamental assumptions:

1. The trait of interest is controlled by the effects of a large number of genes.
2. The effect of each gene is small and roughly equivalent.
3. The environmental effects are randomly distributed among all animals.

Nature of heritability

This equation below is a frank admission by geneticists that genes do not act alone.

Phenotype = genotype + environment (management)

The appearance and ability of a horse is a product of management and training as well as genetics. We expect farm managers to maximize the environment while breeders are responsible for shepherding genes. Yet how do we determine the effects of genetics versus the effects of management? How do we use this information to select desirable traits and to see improvement each generation?

Firstly, we realize that the breeder is actually interested in variation among horses. All horses have heads, run, and perform standard gaits. The presence of one head and four legs is certainly genetic, but is also invariant among horses. Some horses have better heads, some horses run faster, and some horses have smoother gaits than others. The question before the breeder is: "What is the genetic component for the variation in the trait?" Breeders identify, measure, and compare the traits they value among horses.

Second, methods have evolved over the last 100 years to calculate the percentage of observed variation due to genetics (Lynch and Walsh, 1998; Visscher *et al.*, 2008).

The methods begin with measurements of animals and comparisons among related and unrelated animals. Depending on the nature of the data, one of several statistical approaches can be used to estimate heritability from the measurements made.

For dairy cattle, the genetic potential of different bulls to enhance milk production has been measured by studying milk production among thousands of their female offspring out of different cows. For people, the heritability of diseases and other phenotypic traits has been determined by studying large sets of identical and non-identical twins. In every case, the point has been to control the environment, know the relationship among the individuals, and compare the variation as a consequence of the genetic relationships. The quality of the heritability score is influenced by the relationship among the individuals measured, the amount of data collected, and the accuracy of controls for environmental effects, gender, and age. Given the immensity and complexity of the task, the variation among heritability scores from different studies is not surprising.

Variation among phenotypes as a consequence of genetic variation is called heritability. There are two types of heritability: broad-sense heritability and narrow-sense heritability. Broad-sense heritability takes into account all genetic contributions to a trait. These include: genetic influences that act in a cumulative fashion (the additive genetic component – in which, essentially, more is better); the genetic effects that occur when different alleles interact (called the dominance component); the genetic effects from the interactions of genes from different loci (the epistatic component); and any benefits derived from genetic advantage due to the parents, such as milk production by the mother. Broad-sense heritability is very useful for understanding the relative influences of genotype and environment on the phenotype. A large value for broad-sense heritability might imply that changes in management may not be efficacious in affecting the phenotype.

Ironically, the selection of traits based on broad-sense heritability has not been consistently effective. However, whenever a trait shows a high variation for an additive genetic component, selection has been very effective. So the heritability is calculated using just the additive component; this is called the narrow-sense heritability. Narrow-sense heritability has become the primary basis for choosing targets of genetic selection. Whenever the narrow-sense heritability has a value above 0.20, then breeders can anticipate an effective response to selection for that trait. To avoid confusion about the two types of heritability, calculations referring to the broad-sense heritability use the symbol "H^2" while calculations of narrow-sense heritability use the symbol "h^2". When people refer to heritability they are usually referring to its use for selection, and therefore the discussions are about narrow-sense heritability. From this point on, when we refer to heritability, we are referring to narrow-sense heritability.

General observations about heritability

As noted above, the heritability of a trait is characteristic of a population (breed), and values calculated for one breed may not be the same in another. Experiences with different breeds, different species, and different traits indicate the following (Visscher *et al.*, 2008):

1. Measurements of heritability can vary by gender, age, and environment. Accurate heritability measures need to control for these variables.

2. Traits associated with morphology tend to show higher heritability values than those associated with fitness (fertility and survival). This may explain the great success breeders have had in selecting for morphological characteristics such as head shape, conformation, and tail carriage.

3. Many traits show a strong effect of environment on the genetic component, especially morphological traits. For example, various measurements of size have shown high heritability values. However, when individuals are raised in nutrition-restricted environments, the measured heritability value is greatly reduced.

4. Heritability values will not be identical between breeds and species, though they do tend to be similar. If selection is efficacious for a trait in one breed, it is likely to be efficacious in another, although the power of selection may be different.

Heritability estimates for particular traits

Horse racing

The racing performance of horses is well documented. Track locations, distances, times, track conditions, competitors, and money won, as well as pedigrees, are all matters of public record. Breeders have always used such information to make informed but subjective breeding choices – even before the appearance of heritability estimates. The diversity and quality of information provide opportunities and challenges for calculating heritability values. These considerations are reviewed and discussed by Ricard *et al.* (2000) as well as by Langlois (1996). Race time would seem to be an obvious measure of racing performance, except that horses compete over different distances and, often, the official record only includes the winning time. Consequently, some horses that race fail to win and then enter the breeding population without any indication of their genetic value. Finally, with respect to time, horses race against other horses and not against the clock, but achieving a lifetime best for a horse is not a goal for the racehorse owner.

Some advantages exist for comparing horses based on money won in races. In most racing venues, purses are awarded for first, second, and third places; then again, many horses that form part of the breed stock do not win race purses or, conversely, the large prizes from major races skew the distribution of earnings. A heritability calculation is less reliable when large numbers of horses in the breeding population do not have measures of their ability. Langlois (1996) discussed the use of heritabilities for selection in Thoroughbreds, and confirmed that time was not necessarily the best indicator of racing success. He recommended the use of handicapping for the comparison of genetic merit.

Handicapping is one of the most effective methods for comparing horses. Horse racing experts make a subjective evaluation of a horse's racing performance and provide a score called a handicap. The goal of this is to inform racing enthusiasts for the purpose of betting on horse races, but the information has also been used effectively by scientists to estimate heritability values. Gaffney and Cunningham (1988) made use of a handicapping method called the TIMEFORM rating, which is used in the British Isles. The TIMEFORM rating is expressed in terms of the weight that a horse might carry to make its performance close to the population standard. Better horses are assigned more weight. In some ways, this is not unlike the educated judgment of breeders mentioned above. Horses that have not won a race but which have competed will have a TIMEFORM rating.

At the conclusion of their studies, Cunningham's group concluded that the appropriate heritability value for racing performance among Thoroughbreds was 0.36 based on the use of TIMEFORM ratings (Gaffney and Cunningham, 1988). The value of 0.36 implied a moderate-to-high level of heritability and predicted a benefit for selective breeding based on TIMEFORM ratings. This conclusion was reached by consideration of the following considerations. Other heritability values in the literature, including those of the Cunningham group, ranged from less than 0.20 (low heritability) to greater than 0.70 (high heritability); this work is reviewed by Hintz (1980) and Langlois (1980). The variation that was found was a consequence of the different methods used for calculating heritability and biases inherent in the data sets. In practice, breeders and trainers emphasize the stallion in many of their breeding decisions. Therefore, calculations based on relationships among stallions and their offspring, or calculations that compared half sibs of different stallions suffered a bias because: (i) offspring of highly rated stallions received beneficial consideration for racing; and (ii) stallions regarded as having low merit were consistently bred to mares with less merit. Most data came from good stallions and, as a result, the heritability estimates were biased upward (More O'Ferrall and Cunningham, 1976; Langlois, 1980; Ricard et al., 2000).

Overall, the results suggested a moderate heritability (0.34 to 0.36) for racing performance in Thoroughbreds, and a need to control for environmental factors in making calculations (reviewed by Ricard et al., 2000). Carrying the work further, Oki et al. (1997) investigated the heritability of race times based on distances; they found differences for short distances versus long distances, with heritability values higher for short distances. Williamson and Beilharz (1998) developed indices for speed and stamina among Thoroughbreds and noted that speed had a higher heritability than stamina. Later, Tozaki et al. (2011) compared different models for calculating heritability and discussed their uses in light of the discovery of major genes that might confound the assumptions inherent in heritability calculations (for example, MSTN, which is discussed later in the chapter). The value of heritability calculations will increase as we continue to learn about the genetics of racing performance and develop the ability to analyze new sets of data.

Heritability of other horse traits

So far, there has not been extensive use of heritability values for Thoroughbred breeding. However, there has been great interest among the owners of other horse breeds. As noted below, heritability forms the foundation for determining breeding values of individual livestock. Heritability has been measured for other performance traits in horses than racing speed, including drafting ability, gait, jumping, and aspects of dressage; this work is reviewed by Hintz (1980) and by Ricard et al. (2000). Saastamoinen and Barry (2000) have also published an extensive review of heritabilities for conformation and locomotion. In general, heritability for morphological traits was found to be higher than heritability for locomotion and performance traits.

During the last 40 years, programs for the evaluation of sports horses have been established worldwide. These programs have been designed to identify parameters for selection and to determine which animals are superior for transmitting high-quality performance traits to their offspring. Heritabilities have been calculated based on professional evaluations at breed-sanctioned test stations and at competitions. In general, heritabilities calculated based on test station evaluations have been higher than those calculated at competitions. Not all horses compete, so the test stations provide information on more horses and this can be used in determining the heritability of a trait and the breeding value of parents. The use of this type of information has been effective, and improvement has been seen based on these approaches (Viklund *et al.*, 2010). Future challenges are to develop even more effective methods for evaluation, to integrate competition data with field station data, and to standardize evaluations among regions so that the studies can be compared worldwide. The key to making accurate breeding decisions is having quality information in hand.

Estimated Breeding Values (EBV) for Performance Traits

When a trait has a moderate-to-high heritability, we can use the information in making specific breeding decisions. Each individual has a theoretical breeding value, specifically, the genetic contribution that one would expect a parent to make to its offspring. Because we do not fully comprehend the genetics of complex traits, we rely heavily on our knowledge of heritability scores to calculate an estimated breeding value (EBV). The process is as follows: (i) determine the average value for the trait in a population; (ii) measure the value for all offspring of the horse in question in comparison with the other parent; (iii) correlate the values of the trait (e.g. performance or conformation) from the individual and its relatives; and (iv) using the trait heritability, calculate the EBV as the difference in values between the general population and predicted offspring of our horse.

Just as heritability is characteristic of a population at a given point in time, so are EBVs. In other words, as the genetics of a population improve over time as a result of selection, a stallion with a high EBV in 1990 should have a lower EBV value in 2012, reflecting the improved EBV of the breed over that 22 year period.

Árnason and van Vleck (2000) concisely identified the key aspects of horse breeding that make the use of EBV important and effective for horses:

1. Pedigrees are available for many generations for many breeds of horse.
2. Important traits are measured in both males and females for use in selection.
3. Horses may not express the performance trait until maturity.
4. The horse has a long generation interval (10–12 years).
5. Horses have a long period of fertility, with some being reproductively active for more than 15 years.
6. Selective breeding is the general practice, thus making it relatively easy to determine the heritability of traits.
7. There are large differences in the economic value of horses based on their assumed genetic merit.

In summary, the quality of the information available makes genetic selection feasible; the long gestation length makes methodical approaches desirable; and the long fertility period of individual horses makes the calculations valuable.

Best linear unbiased prediction (BLUP)

A system called best linear unbiased prediction (BLUP) has been successful for making genetic improvement in other livestock. BLUP was proposed for use with horses in the 1970s (Langlois *et al.*, 1975; Minkema, 1976). In those studies, the scientists considered how BLUP might be used to predict which horses would make superior breeding stock to improve racing performance in trotters. Today, BLUP is used to evaluate everything, including conformation, gait, and character.

The first actual use of BLUP to determine EBV was reported by Árnason (1980) to evaluate gait for Icelandic horses. The method has evolved into a very sophisticated system of evaluation for a wide range of traits. Breeders can access records to determine the EBVs for many different traits. For example, one trait valued by breeders of Icelandic horses is the gait "tölt", sometimes referred to as a "running walk". Breeders have agreed on a scoring system for this trait. In this example, consider that an average value might be a score of 7.3 in the year 2010. BLUP is used to evaluate the population at large using all the available information, including evaluation of the horse at hand, of the parents, and of all available offspring. The more information that is available, the more accurate the assessment will be. The population is considered to have a normal distribution for the trait (simple additive genetics), with a mean score transformed to a value of 100. A horse with a score of 100 is not expected to improve the performance of its offspring above the population mean. A stallion with a score of 110 and a mare with a score of 90 would cancel each other out and produce an offspring that would, on average, perform at the population mean. Mating a mare with a BLUP score of 90 for tölt to a stallion with a BLUP score of 120 would be predicted to produce an offspring that would perform 10% above the population mean for genetic gain.

Clearly, the effectiveness of BLUP scores for calculating EBV depends on the amount of information available for each horse, the quality of the calculated heritability values for each trait, and the veracity of the measures. Sometimes, or perhaps often, information will be incomplete or compromised in some fashion. Therefore, confidence level for the EBV needs to be considered along with the actual EBV score. Stallions with lots of offspring will have more accurate EBVs than mares or stallions with fewer offspring. In any case, the BLUP score for EBV provides a rational approach to selection. We can anticipate continued improvement in the system as more records are compiled, and computer programs are developed to account for the various nuances that we discover for performance.

These approaches are also being used widely by Warmblood horse registries (Hanoverian, Holsteiner, Oldenburg, Trakehner, Dutch Warmblood, Swedish Warmblood, Selle Français, etc.) to aid in the improvement of sports horses. Extensive programs have been established for compiling records of horses at test stations – independent of competitions – to determine an EBV for horses in the breeding population. The method is an effective approach to controlling for environmental variation in calculating EBVs as well as providing performance evaluations on horses even when they are not chosen for competition.

Genetic Markers for Traits

So far, we have considered the genetics of performance without considering any actual genes. Heritability and EBV are mathematical constructs of the genome. Molecular geneticists investigate the contribution of individual genes to performance. Since the completion of the horse whole genome sequence, scientists have determined that horses have approximately 21,000 genes and 2.47 billion bases of DNA. Relating specific genes to performance could be valuable for horse breeders. However, simply having the whole genome sequence has not made this a simple task. Scientists have begun using the approaches described in Chapter 3 to study genes and performance.

There are two major reasons to study the molecular genetics of performance. Firstly, heritability only deals with the additive aspects of genetics; it ignores epigenetics, interactions between genes, and the interactions of genes with environment. As we achieve maximal genetic improvement using the additive genetics of this infinitesimal model, the other aspects of genetics become more important. Molecular genetic approaches will provide additional tools.

Second, a major problem with the use of BLUP and EBVs is that it takes a relatively long time to determine the breeding value of a horse. The genetic merit for an individual is highly speculative until it actually performs, and is unknown until it actually produces offspring. Through the process of evaluation, some horses are to be judged useful for genetic improvement, while others are rejected. A trainer/breeder begins with a large group of horses, gradually culling those that are judged to be inadequate. This process is both time-consuming and costly.

Marker assisted selection (MAS)

An approach called marker assisted selection (MAS) could be a benefit for breeders. MAS entails the discovery of a genetic marker associated with a desirable trait, and enabling the selection of individuals based largely on the presence or absence of that genetic marker. The genetic marker may be a DNA microsatellite (see Chapter 11), a SNP (see Chapter 3), or even a protein product of a gene. We may not know the precise gene or genetic basis for the trait, but if the genetic marker is close to a DNA feature responsible for the trait, we can use the genetic marker as a proxy for that gene. The goal of MAS is to use genetic typing at birth to identify horses that have potential to be superior performers. Horses that are rejected based on MAS can be used for other activities, and avoid the frustration for horse and horse owner of trying find talent that does not exist. The costs for horse owners are less and the time required to make genetic gain can be reduced by identifying and including superior individuals earlier on in the breeding programs.

MAS requires the discovery of genes or genetic markers that are associated with performance traits. Genes that have an impact on complex traits such as performance traits are called quantitative trait loci (QTLs). We assume that many QTLs will exist for complex traits, but a few will have a major impact on the trait, making them readily recognizable in genetic studies. The tools created in connection with the whole genome sequencing of the horse have made it possible to investigate performance at the genome level. The first target has been the study of racing performance.

Major gene for racing performance: *MSTN*

A QTL for Thoroughbred racing has been identified on ECA18 very close to the myostatin gene (*MSTN*) (Binns *et al.*, 2010; Hill *et al.*, 2010a; Tozaki *et al.*, 2010).

Myostatin is a protein that limits the differentiation and growth of skeletal muscles. Cattle with mutations in this gene produce more muscle and are popularly referred to as "double-muscled" because of their very muscular appearance. A mutation that destroyed the function of this gene was associated with superior sprinting ability in whippet dogs (Mosher *et al.*, 2007). Based on this observation, Hill *et al.* (2010a) investigated a genetic marker (SNP) associated with *MSTN* that that was strongly associated with best race distance among elite Thoroughbred racehorses. For the SNP sequence variant g.66493737C>T (in which the base C can be substituted by T), winners of sprinting races were most likely to possess only the SNP variant with C (designated "C"), winners of distance races were most likely to possess only the SNP variant with T (designated "T"), while winners of middle distance races were reported to have both "C" and "T". The location of the SNP fell outside the DNA coding region for the myostatin protein, and no mutation or variant was discovered that altered the structure or integrity of the protein. Mosher *et al.* (2007) speculated that this mutation, or another outside the coding sequence of the gene, regulated the expression of the racing phenotype. Their work was confirmed in two similar studies of horses, although different markers were implicated (Binns *et al.*, 2010; Tozaki *et al.*, 2010). In further work by Hill *et al.* (2010b), a genome-wide SNP association study was performed for optimum racing distance in elite Thoroughbred horses. This confirmed that the g.66493737C>T SNP was the superior sequence variant in the prediction of distance aptitude in racehorses.

Based on the physiology of the racing performance trait, its association with the *MSTN* chromosome region, and the observation of a similar effect for dogs, it seems likely that the effect of the g.66493737C>T SNP is due to *MSTN*. The precise mutation has not yet been found, but the C and T SNPs identified in these studies are so strongly associated with the trait that breeders can use them in their selection programs. Further evidence for the efficacy of this QTL comes from studies of other horse breeds. Bower *et al.* (2012) showed that the *MSTN* allele with the T SNP was most common allele among Arabian horses prized for endurance, while the *MSTN* allele C SNP was most common among American Quarter Horses selected for sprinting ability (Table 14.1). Based on an extensive survey of horses from around the world, and of equids of different species, Bower *et al.* concluded that the original form of the gene was for the endurance type (T SNP), and that the sprint form of the gene (C SNP) likely appeared later and has been subject to selection among racing breeds.

Table 14.1. Frequency of the myostatin gene (*MSTN*) mutation ("C" or "T" SNP) among horses of different breeds (adapted from Bower *et al.*, 2012).

Breed	Use	Number	C SNP	T SNP
Egyptian Arabian	Endurance	30	0.08	0.92
Icelandic horse	Gaited	21	0.17	0.83
Quarter Horse	Sprinter	35	0.90	0.10
Standardbred	1 mile	63	0.00	1.00
Thoroughbred	Distance	96	0.34	0.66
Thoroughbred	Sprinter	69	0.70	0.30
Donkey	Other species	40	0.00	1.00

Bower *et al.* (2012) note that this is only the beginning of the discovery of QTLs for racing performance. These studies also showed that other genetic and management factors are important. A fruitful approach to discovering other performance genes would be to investigate successful sprinters that do not have the C SNP and successful endurance horses that do not have the T SNP. Other, as yet unidentified, genes than *MSTN* may play a role for these horses, and although the QTL for *MSTN* is a valuable tool for breeders, it does not replace testing on the track. Future research in this area will focus on the discovery of additional QTLs as well as on investigations of training and management techniques for horses with different QTLs.

Major gene for gait: *DMRT3*

The standard three gaits for horses are walk, trot, and canter/gallop. However, horses have been prized and selected for the ability to perform other gaits. Specifically, these are the pace and a high-speed four-beat gait that varies between breeds and has been called amble, the running walk, tölt, rack, stepping pace, fox trot, single foot, or paso gait (Harris, 1993). Genetics and training influence gait. Andersson *et al.* (2012) have reported the first gene that has a major impact on gait. They used molecular genetic techniques to map, locate, and sequence the Doublesex- and mab-3-related transcription factor 3 gene (*DMRT3*) to identify a mutation that disrupts gene function and is common among pacing horses, racing trotters and four-beat gaited horses. They tested a wide range of breeds, and obtained the results shown in Table 14.2. The frequency distribution of the mutation in *DMRT3* suggests that the gene is advantageous for horses performing more than the three basic gaits (gaited horses), but is disadvantageous for others. The gene was absent in the non-gaited horses but common or fixed among gaited and harness racing breeds.

The results for racing trotters seem unusual because the *DMRT3* trait was identified as being associated with pacing or with four-beat gaits, and the trot is considered a two-beat gait. Racing trotters are asked to trot at high speeds, well above those at which most horses would break into a gallop. In this way, they are asked to perform the gait in an unusual fashion and may even depart from precisely performing a "hard, two-beat trot".

There are likely to be additional genes influencing gaits. Even though Icelandic horses are all gaited, they exhibited considerable genetic variation for *DMRT3*. Likewise, the differences in performance among gaited horses, pacers, and racing trotters suggests greater genetic complexity. Those genes may be major genes like *DMRT3*, or the genetic effect may be the result of a large number of different genes, each with a small effect.

These studies provide some of the first molecular tests for predicting aspects of performance. Future work is certain to lead to discoveries of genes influencing other performance traits. While development of these predictive tests is exciting, the long-term goals of this work are to: (i) identify the physiological basis underlying superior performance; (ii) determine what genotypes are suitable for which activities; and (iii) determine how to tailor management and training programs to obtain optimum performance from each horse.

Table 14.2. Gene frequency for the *DMRT3* mutation among different horse breeds (adapted from Andersson *et al.*, 2012).

Breed	Number	Mutation
Gaited horses		
Fox Trotter	40	0.95
Icelandic horses		
Four-gaited	124	0.65
Pacing	66	0.99
Kentucky Mountain	22	0.95
Paso Fino	45	1.00
Peruvian Paso	19	1.00
Rocky Mountain	17	1.00
Tennessee Walker	33	0.98
Non-gaited horses		
Arabian	18	0.00
Gotland pony	28	0.00
North-Swedish Draft	31	0.00
Przewalski	6	0.00
Swedish Ardennes	22	0.00
Swedish Warmblood	64	0.00
Thoroughbred	29	0.00
Harness racing horses		
Pacer (USA)	40	1.00
Trotter (France)	47	0.77
Trotter (Sweden)	270	0.97
Trotter (USA)	57	1.00

References

Andersson, L.S. *et al.* (2012) Mutations in *DMRT3* affect locomotion in horses and spinal circuit function in mice. *Nature* 488, 642–646.

Árnason, T. (1980) Genetic studies on the Icelandic Toelter-horse (estimation of breeding values). Paper presented at: *31st Annual Meeting of the European Association for Animal Production, September 1–4, 1980*. Commission on Horse Production, Munich, Germany, p. 5.

Arnason [Árnason], T. and van Vleck, L.D. (2000) Genetic improvement of the horse. In: Bowling, A.T. and Ruvinsky, A. (eds) *The Genetics of the Horse*. CAB International, Wallingford, UK, pp. 473–498.

Binns, M.M., Boehler, D.A. and Lambert, D.H. (2010) Identification of the myostatin locus (*MSTN*) as having a major effect on optimum racing distance in the Thoroughbred horse in the USA. *Animal Genetics* 41 (Supplement 2), 154–158.

Bower, M.A. *et al.* (2012) The genetic origin and history of speed in the Thoroughbred racehorse. *Nature Communications* 3, 643.

Gaffney, B. and Cunningham, E.P. (1988) Estimation of genetic trend in racing performance of Thoroughbred horses. *Nature* 332, 722–724.

Harris, S.E. (1993) *Horse Gaits, Balance and Movement*. Simon and Schuster, New York.

Hill, E.W., Gu, J., Eivers, S.S., Fonseca, R.G., McGivney, B.A., Govindarajan, P., Orr, N., Katz, L.M. and MacHugh, D.E. (2010a) A sequence polymorphism in *MSTN* predicts sprinting ability and racing stamina in Thoroughbred horses. *PLoS One* 5(1): e8645, doi: 10.1371/journal.pone.0008645.

Hill, E.W., McGivney, B.A., Gu, J., Whiston, R. and MacHugh, D.E. (2010b) A genome-wide SNP-association study confirms a sequence variant (g.66493737C>T) in the equine myostatin (*MSTN*) gene as the most powerful predictor of optimum racing distance for Thoroughbred racehorses. *BMC Genomics* 11: 552, doi:10.1186/1471-2164-11-552.

Hintz, H.F. (1980) Genetics of performance in the horse. *Journal of Animal Science* 51, 582–594.

Langlois, B. (1980) Heritability of racing ability in Thoroughbreds – a review. *Livestock Production Science* 7, 591–605.

Langlois, B. (1996) A consideration of the genetic aspects of some current practices in Thoroughbred horse breeding. *Annales de Zootechnie* 45, 41–51.

Langlois, B., Poirel, D., Tastu, D. and Rose, J. (1975) Analyse statistique et génétique des gains des *pur sang anglais* de trois ans dans les courses plates françaises [Statistical analysis and genetic gains of three year old English thoroughbreds in French flat races]. *Annales de Génétique et de Selection Animale* 7, 387–408.

Lynch, M. and Walsh, B. (1998) *Genetics and Analysis of Quantitative Traits*. Sinauer Associates, Sunderland, Massachusetts.

Minkema, D. (1976) Studies on the genetics of trotting performance in Dutch trotters. II. A method for the breeding value estimation of trotter stallions. *Annales de Génétique et de Selection Animale* 8, 511–526.

More O'Ferrall, G.J. and Cunningham, E.P. (1974) Heritability of racing performance in Thoroughbred horses. *Livestock Production Science* 1, 87–97.

Mosher, D.S., Quignon, P., Bustamante, C.D., Sutter, N.B., Mellersh, C.S., Parker, H.G. and Ostrander, E.A. (2007) A mutation in the myostatin gene increases muscle mass and enhances racing performance in heterozygote dogs. *PLoS Genetics* 3(5): e79, doi:10.1371/journal.pgen.0030079.

Oki, H., Sasaki, Y. and Willham, R.L. (1997) Estimation of genetic correlations between racing times recorded at different racing distances by restricted maximum likelihood in Thoroughbred racehorses. *Journal of Animal Breeding and Genetics* 114, 185–189.

Ricard, A., Bruns, E. and Cunningham, E.P. (2000) Genetics of performance traits. In: Bowling, A.T. and Ruvinsky, A. (eds) *The Genetics of the Horse*. CAB International, Wallingford, UK, pp. 411–438.

Saastamoinen, M.T. and Barrey, E. (2000) Genetics of conformation, locomotion and physiological traits. In: Bowling, A.T. and Ruvinsky, A. (eds) *The Genetics of the Horse*. CAB International, Wallingford, UK, pp. 439–472.

Tozaki, T., Miyake, T., Kakoi, H., Gawahara, H., Sugita, S., Hasegawa, T., Ishida, N., Hirota, K. and Nakano, Y. (2010) A genome-wide association study for racing performances in Thoroughbreds clarifies a candidate region near the *MSTN* gene. *Animal Genetics* 41 (Supplement 2), 28–35.

Viklund, Å., Näsholm, A., Strandberg, E. and Philipsson, J. (2010) Effects of long-time series of data on genetic evaluations for performance of Swedish Warmblood riding horses. *Animal* 4, 1823–1831.

Visscher, P.M., Hill, W.G. and Wray, N.R. (2008) Heritability in the genomics era – concepts and misconceptions. *Nature Reviews Genetics* 9, 255–266.

Williamson, S.A. and Beilharz, R.G. (1998) The inheritance of speed, stamina and other racing performance characters in the Australian Thoroughbred. *Journal of Animal Breeding and Genetics* 115, 1–16.

15 Pedigrees and Breeding Schemes

Breeders cannot change Mendelian genetics, nor the number of genes involved in traits, nor their linkage relationships. They cannot change the physiological interactions of gene products, but they can hope through selective mating to produce gene combinations that consistently result in high-quality stock.

Establishing Pedigrees

The formation of breed societies to record animal pedigrees – the foundation of western livestock breeding practices, traces to England in the early 19th century. Breed societies aimed to protect and promote a distinctive animal type that was consistently superior in production or performance characteristics compared with common stock. The achievements of these societies lent credence to the notion that "pure" stock, whose genealogy was faithfully recorded and published, was highly desirable for successful animal breeding. The availability of recorded pedigrees, presumably authentic, led to attempts to use them to correlate success with pedigree patterns, and as a tool to predict the outcome of matings.

Broadly speaking the systems of mating that a breeder may choose are:

1. mating like to like (based on pedigree likeness or individual likeness, such as performance success, disposition or body shape)
2. random mating (no selection)
3. mating unlike to unlike (based on outcrossed pedigrees or individual extremes, such as tall with short, or rangy with compact, or hot temperament with mellow).

Successful examples of all these schemes could be cited for any breed. Every horse breeder needs to understand the genetic principles underlying these situations and then to decide which is the most appropriate for each breeding pair.

This chapter discusses terms and concepts of pedigree study. One aim of teaching is to encourage debate and critical examination of issues and statements. This chapter challenges some of the myths of horse breeding. If it provokes discussion and sound research to help breeders make wise choices, it will have served one of its intended purposes. For additional discussion, consult Lush (1945), a classic, clearly written animal breeding text.

The pedigree format: the standard diagram

We use pedigrees to help us understand what genes a horse might have. Mostly, what we can learn from a pedigree provides us with a subjective impression, although some "real" genetic information can be learned. For example, a tobiano horse has no possibility of being homozygous for tobiano if it does not have both a tobiano sire and a tobiano dam. Notice, however, that if the tobiano does have two tobiano parents, the pedigree cannot tell us whether the offspring has one or two tobiano alleles.

The routine (standard) pedigree format is a diagram of a "begat" listing. By convention, the offspring is named to the left of the page and the first column to the right lists the parents, arranged with the sire at the top (Fig. 15.1). The next column gives the parents of the parents (the grandparents of the offspring), and so on. The pedigree may be a listing of names, or names and registration numbers, or may also include year of birth, coat color, breeder, photographs, and outstanding performance records. The more information provided, the more accurate will be any estimation of an individual's characteristics.

Relatedness and "percentage of blood"

Offspring resemble their parents to varying degrees, but the proportional genetic contribution of each parent is constant: half the genes of an offspring come from the mother and half from the father (except for the mitochondrial genes that are maternally inherited in a non-Mendelian fashion). A relatedness coefficient of 50% or 0.5 is assigned to the parent–offspring relationship.

Full siblings *on average* share 50% of their genes. For every locus, assuming the parents are heterozygous for different alleles, the offspring have four possible allelic combinations: 25% of the time they will have received the same alleles from their dam; 25% of the time they will have received the same alleles from their sire; 25% of the time they will have received no alleles in common from sire or dam; and 25% of the time they will have received the same alleles from both sire and dam. The random assortment of chromosome pairs during gamete formation means that we cannot predict the exact proportion of genes that any two full siblings have in common; we can only provide an average value for all genes of full siblings as a group. In practical terms, and stallion advertisements to the contrary, one cannot assume that a full brother to a proven stallion will be an equivalently successful sire. Certainly, he has a greater likelihood of sharing genes with the proven stallion than he does with

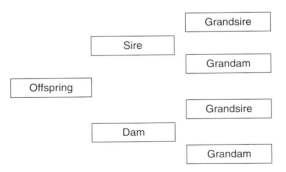

Fig. 15.1. Conventional pedigree format, providing a short listing of the parents and grandparents of a particular offspring. A typical pedigree will provide five or six prior generations, rather than the two given here. The more information provided about each of the ancestors, the more useful will be the pedigree for predicting the potential of the offspring.

a non-relative, but there is no guarantee that he has received the group of genes that sets his brother apart from the rest of the breed.

Half-siblings on average share 25% of their genes, and first cousins share about 12.5%. Relatedness decreases by half with each succeeding generation. More complicated relationships can easily be calculated.

In the simplest of pedigree evaluations, breeders may talk about "percentage of blood". Of course, blood is not a unit of inheritance, but is used in this context to imply genetic traits. Summing the relatedness coefficients for every occurrence of particular ancestors in the pedigree provides the proportion by source of an individual's genes (see Fig. 15.2). The sum is not an exact proportion, but a statement of the most likely percentage. It is always possible that the gene proportion could be larger or smaller than the calculated relatedness coefficient.

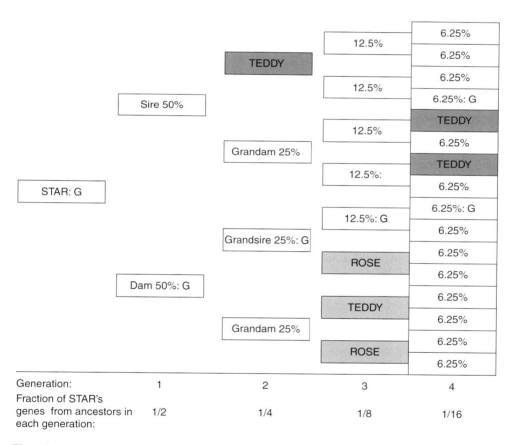

Generation:	1	2	3	4
Fraction of STAR's genes from ancestors in each generation:	1/2	1/4	1/8	1/16

Fig. 15.2. The fraction of an individual's genes most likely to come from each ancestor is presented in this conventional pedigree format. For a hypothetical case, consider the calculation of a pedigree for STAR. Summing the fractions, this pedigree could be described as "50% TEDDY", meaning that *on* average an individual with this pedigree could be expected to have 50% of its genes derived from TEDDY, but could also have a smaller or a larger proportion. STAR has a relatedness coefficient of 25% to the mare ROSE. Horses of gray color are designated with G.

Evaluation of pedigree influences

A four- to five-generation pedigree with its 30–62 names among the various generations can be intimidating to newcomers to whom few of the names have any recognition value. It is natural to seek simple rules to reduce the blur of names to a meaningful collection. Some breeders believe that horses beyond the fourth generation in a pedigree need not be considered. This statement is usually given to justify the unimportance of pedigree elements generally considered unfavorably. Other breeders use pedigrees as "witch hunts" and will not use a horse whose pedigree has *any* perceived undesirable element. Usually, this thinking is associated with trying to avoid genetic diseases that are associated with named horses. The balanced view of pedigree evaluation does not use simple generalizations, but requires thoughtful analysis on a case-by-case basis.

The genome of any horse is always a composite of contributions from the entire pedigree. The fraction of genes in an offspring's genome attributed to particular ancestors in distant generations is small. Any single gene in a fifth generation ancestor has only about a 3% chance of passing through all the meiotic partitions and arriving in the genome of the great-great-great grandchild. Yet consider a pedigree from the standpoint of a single color gene, such as gray, which can be easily traced through a pedigree. In the pedigree illustrated (Fig. 15.2), STAR is a gray, with two potential pedigree sources of the dominant allele G. The gray horse on the sire's side (indicated by "G") cannot be the source of STAR's gray color, because the color is not even transmitted from that gray ancestor to the next generation. The gray ancestor on the dam's side, which is traceable from one generation to the next, is clearly the source of the gray color for STAR. With every generation, the G on the dam's side had a 50% chance of being lost from this pedigree, but in each case it was transmitted forward. The gray color example shows it is not the position in the pedigree that determines whether traits are transmitted, it is the chance events of probability.

Relate this color example to genes that are not shown on a pedigree, say disease genes. Among ancestors in the same generation with the same heterozygous pair of alleles for a given gene, it may be very difficult to determine which of their allelic alternatives was transmitted when their presence is not phenotypically obvious. A single disease or color gene could be traceable to a sole source in each generation. Conversely, multiple elements could be possible sources of the gene. If a trait is known *not* to have been transmitted to the next generation, it is a waste of time to continue to consider that individual or pedigree line as a source of the given desirable (or undesirable) gene.

Inbreeding, Linebreeding, Outcrossing, and Assortative Mating

Inbreeding and linebreeding

Inbreeding pairs related animals, such as father and daughter, mother and son, brother and sister, or cousins. STAR (Fig. 15.2) and his sire are inbred to TEDDY. STAR'S dam is inbred to the mare ROSE, but STAR is not inbred to her, because she does not occur on both sides of his pedigree.

Linebreeding is the term used by breeders to describe their breeding programs based on multiple pedigree crosses to a single exceptional animal. STAR is linebred to the "highly renowned" TEDDY.

An inbreeding coefficient, F, provides a probability that the alleles in any gene pair will be *identical by descent* (homozygous) from an ancestor found on both the sire's and dam's sides of the offspring's pedigree. Examples of F values for matings in human pedigree terms are: parent–offspring or full sibs (0.25); uncle–niece (0.125); first cousins (0.0625); second cousins (0.016). STAR's F value is 0.09375, meaning about 9% of his genes would be homozygous for alleles originating from TEDDY. Several inbred relationships may occur within a horse pedigree. In those cases, an inbreeding coefficient is calculated by summing the coefficients of all the relationships.

In general in horse breeding programs, calculation of inbreeding coefficients probably contributes little of practical value. For intensely inbred breeding groups in which the immediate aim is to select matings to maintain a maximum of genetic diversity (say, for an endangered species), selection for lower inbreeding coefficients could be useful for choosing among breeding pair options. Readers interested in learning to calculate such values using examples of horses may want to consult van Vleck (1990).

Toward homozygosity

Inbreeding not only increases the proportion of genes that trace to a given ancestor, it also increases the likelihood that the genes will be homozygous. The premise under-lying the positive attitude toward inbreeding is that homozygosity is desirable, but these genes may *not* have been homozygous in the admired ancestor. Key components for working with inbred pedigrees to avoid producing foals homozygous for an unde-sirable trait include accurate tests to identify trait carriers and knowledge of basic genetics. For example, inbreeding to a palomino Quarter Horse stallion, highly esteemed for his conformation as well as color, could lead to the production of cre-mello foals that would not be eligible for registration regardless of desirable confor-mation and quality. Breeders could avoid the cremello problem and still inbreed to a palomino source if they apply the principles of coat color genetics and select appro-priate breeding pairs (i.e. avoid breeding together palominos, buckskins, or their combination). This example illustrates the possibilities of using basic genetics to avoid producing foals homozygous for an undesirable trait while working with het-erozygous (carrier) pedigrees.

Although physical uniformity may be a goal of purebred breeding programs, extreme genetic uniformity is probably not desirable, because hardiness, vigor, and reproductive soundness may decrease with increasing homozygosity. In a study of fertility and inbreeding in Standardbreds, reproductive performance was not affected at the low inbreeding levels of 7–10% typically encountered in domestic horse breed-ing programs (Cothran *et al.*, 1984). The effects of high levels of inbreeding on domes-tic horse fertility have not been reported.

Genetic alternatives will become restricted as homozygosity increases in any inbred group. Inbreeding tends to create distinctive breeding groups through chance "fixing" of genes. If several breeders undertake inbreeding programs independent of each others' stock, different genes can become fixed in each group, even though their genetic repertories might initially have been quite similar. Within a larger (breed) context, diversity can be maintained by establishing several inbred lines.

Closed stud books

Many stud books have regulations that prevent the use of animals outside the registry, effectively creating a closed gene pool. The aim of this closure is to encourage breeding of a consistent type of stock with excellence for a selected set of breed characteristics. For closed stud books, the gene pool is initially defined by variants provided by the founder stock. With a sufficiently large founder population and no historical periods of severely restricted population size (bottlenecks), the gene pool may be quite diverse, and new gene combinations may still be realized for tens of generations.

In this case, the only sources of new genetic material will be mutation or undetected crossbreeding (gene introgression). The mutation process occurs spontaneously and continuously, but most mutations are immediately eliminated because they are deleterious to the organism, or they are eliminated within a few generations by random chance. The introduction of new genetic material into a closed stud book through crossbreeding can be avoided by denying registration to horses that fail parentage verification tests.

The maintenance of diversity may be an appropriate breeding goal, particularly within the context of a closed breeding program. Several horse breeds are fractionated into subsets of inbred lines, sometimes defended so vehemently by their protagonists that personal feuding between owners of different substrains becomes surprisingly intense and bitter. The far-sighted view of breed promotion recognizes the value of maintaining multiple lines to preserve diversity for the genetic health of the breed.

Inbreeding in short versus long pedigrees

Owners generally see no more than a five- or six-generation pedigree of their animals, owing perhaps to constraints as trivial as paper size for printing pedigrees, but also to the time necessary to research and write out more generations. If distant generations could be viewed as easily on paper as the more immediate ones, breeders might be surprised to find out to how few founders their purebred animals trace from. In a study of inbreeding and pedigree structure in Standardbred horses, MacCluer *et al.* (1983) determined that inbreeding coefficients calculated from 27-generation pedigrees (back to breed founders) were increased by nearly 2.4 times (from 0.0375 to 0.0888) compared with those calculated from the conventional short pedigrees usually considered by breeders.

Outcrossing

In contrast to inbreeding or linebreeding schemes, some breeders use outcrossing programs to meet their goals. Outcrossing means the breeding together of unrelated animals. Outcrossing in the context of a closed breed is practiced by avoiding or minimizing the duplication of names in pedigrees, although it is likely that the animals are related in distant generations.

Some breeds allow the use of outcrossing with horses not in their stud books, but usually only to selected breeds that are considered important sources for obtaining or maintaining performance or conformation characteristics. In theory, horses that are the products of outcrossing (also called crossbreeding) programs may be more heterozygous than inbred horses. Crossbreds might be outstanding performers, but as breeding stock inconsistently pass on their desirable characteristics. Warmblood breeds use outcrossing extensively – in combination with performance testing schemes – to maintain a breeding stock pool that is strongly selected for a subset of traits associated with predictable excellence in 3 day events and selected specialties.

Assortative mating

Mating like to like on the basis of their perceived similarities, without regard to pedigree, is called positive assortative mating. This technique can combine animals with similar genes or animals with different genes that manifest a similar phenotype. In any case, the goal is to produce an animal that closely resembles the parents.

Mating together animals of unlike phenotypes is called negative assortative mating. The goal of this process is to breed offspring that are not as extreme as either parent. The consideration of pedigrees from the standpoint of whether they represent positive or negative assortative matings can be useful for thinking about individual traits, but probably has limited application in the context of the overall horse. A racehorse breeder would probably select positive assortative mating for speed (e.g. mating a sprinter to sprinter or distance winner to a distance winner), but negative assortative mating if seeking to overcome conformation defects (e.g. mating to a heavier boned mate to a improve light-boned animal). Most matings combine positive assortative mating for some traits with negative assortative mating for others, but in practice breeders seldom articulate their breeding decisions in such terms.

Tail-male and tail-female lineages

Tail-male lineage

Breeders may classify breeding lines by a tail-male pedigree lineage that traces the top line of a conventionally drawn pedigree back to a noted founder stallion. In Fig. 15.3,

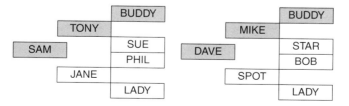

Fig. 15.3. SAM, TONY, DAVE and MIKE share tail-male lineage and a Y chromosome from the stallion BUDDY.

this is BUDDY. Clustering male horses based on their shared tail-male relationship makes biological sense in the light of transmission of the Y chromosome from male to male. These horses necessarily share the few genes present on the Y chromosome (barring the effects of recombination and mutation).

From a genetic standpoint, it is not clear how females could be considered to have a connection to a tail-male group because they do not have the founder Y chromosome. After several generations, both males and females may have no autosomal genes remaining from that founder source.

Tail-female lineage, strain breeding and families

Several meanings are associated with the terms strain and family when applied to pedigree relationships. Probably the most common use for either term (and they may be used interchangeably) is for a group of animals selectively bred for several generations from a subset of animals within a breed. This usage often reflects the long-standing successful breeding program of a particular stable, stud farm, or group of cooperative breeders.

A different meaning is attached to these terms by some Thoroughbred and Arabian horse breeders, who tie physical and mental traits to tail-female pedigree connections. In Fig. 15.4, the founder mare is LADY. Bruce Lowe, an Australian who made extensive studies of Thoroughbred pedigrees, developed a system for predicting racing excellence based on tail-female founders (Bruce Lowe families). The Bedouin Arab used the tail-female convention to describe the relationship of their horses to celebrated foundation mares (strains), a tradition that is still continued by some breeders.

The performance excellence of horses sharing tail-female connections could be based on maternal inheritance through mitochondria, but any such relationship between performance traits and specific mitochondrial genes currently awaits validation. Some breeders strive for multiple generations of breeding within the same strain (sires and dams of the same strain), but the underlying biological basis for attaining excellence in this way is not clear.

A tail-female connection among female horses is not chromosomally analogous to the Y chromosome sharing among males with a tail-male relationship. Any grandchild of our hypothetical LADY in Fig. 15.4 has only a 50% chance of receiving one of LADY's X chromosomes. Two otherwise unrelated granddaughters (or grandsons) have only a 12.5% chance of receiving the same X chromosome from their common maternal grandmother. Thus, the persistence of traits through pedigrees cannot be routinely traced to X chromosome sharing from a tail-female connection.

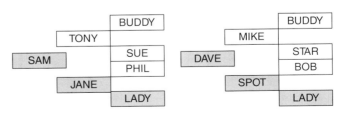

Fig. 15.4. SAM, JANE, DAVE and SPOT share tail-female lineage to the mare LADY.

Questioning Breeding Myths in the Light of Genetics

Newcomers to horse breeding often look for pedigree formulas or hope to emulate a particular breeder's program by using related stock. Unfortunately for novices, the truths of horse breeding are that many successful horse breeding judgments are in equal measure luck and intuition. Horse breeding is not as easy to fit to formulas as breeding for meat or milk production. Many of the highly valued traits of horses, such as breed type or "way of going", are subjectively evaluated in show ring events. Winners may reflect the skills and show ring savvy of the trainer/handler, as much as it does the innate abilities of the horse. Some breeders can learn to predict to their satisfaction the approximate phenotype to expect from a selected mating because of their years of experience in studying horses and their pedigrees, but their skills cannot always be taught to others and may not work with unfamiliar pedigrees.

Nicks

Horses considered to be of excellent quality often present a pattern of recurring pedigree elements. Breeders naturally seek to define pedigree formulas or "nicks" to design matings that will consistently replicate this quality. However, breeding horses is not like following a recipe to make a cake. You cannot precisely measure or direct the ingredients (genes) of the pedigree mixture as you can the flour, sugar, chocolate, eggs, and baking powder for a cake. You can construct pedigrees to look very similar *on paper*, but the individuals described by those pedigrees may be phenotypically (and genetically) quite different. Before seriously considering any breeding formula scheme it is essential that breeders understand the most basic lesson of genetics, that *each mating will produce a genetically different individual with a new combination of genes*.

A certain nick is often expressed as cross of stallion A with stallion B – an obvious impossibility! Probably one source of this convention is that it is easier to become familiar with the characteristics of the offspring of stallions than mares, because they usually have a great number of foals. Another source is the perceived need to reduce complex pedigrees to an easily described summary. Breeding stallion A to the *daughters* of stallion B (this would be the genetically correct description of some nicks) may produce horses of a relatively consistent type compared with the rest of the breed. For mares of the next generation, the "magic" nick (stallion C) is again at the mercy of genetic mechanisms that assure genes are constantly reassorted with every individual and every generation. Some breeders are reluctant to introduce stallion C at all, preferring to continue with their A–B horses, breeding their A–B mares to A–B stallions. If a nick works, and it can appear to do so for some breeders, basic understanding of genetics tells us that it is seldom a long-term, multigenerational proposition unless it is guided by an astute breeder who is making breeding decisions on individual characteristics, and not merely the paper pedigrees.

Basing a program on champions

Novice breeders are often counseled to "start with a good mare". This seems to be reasonable advice, but does not make it clear that the critical point is learning to recognize a good mare. Sometimes, breeders fail to produce a foal that matches the quality of its excellent dam, while less impressive mares in other programs produce successfully. Probably the lack of objective criteria for evaluating horses accounts for both observations. A "good mare" need not be a champion, and a champion is not guaranteed by dint of show ribbons to be a "good mare". In addition, we do not know the inheritance patterns of highly valued traits for show ring excellence. If the ideal type is generated by heterozygosity (e.g. the ever useful example of palomino), the only infallible way to produce foals that meet the criterion of excellence (palomino color) is to use parents of less desirable type (chestnuts bred to cremellos). This example is not to be taken as a general license to use horses of inferior quality, but to provoke critical thinking about the adequacy of general breeding formulas to guide specific programs.

Other breeders pride themselves in structuring programs based on using exceptional stallions. However, breeders should be aware of the fallacy of this type of strategy: "I like stallion Y but I can't afford the risk to breed my mare to an unknown stallion like Y – I can only breed to a National Champion like Z". Any breeding is at risk of producing a less than perfect foal, but the advertising hyperbole leads novices to think that certain avenues are practically foolproof. Included in the best thought out breeding plans must be an appreciation of the ever-present potential of deleterious genes being included with those that are highly prized. It is irresponsible to assume that an animal is without undesirable genes. The wise breeder understands the task as minimizing the risk of creating a foal with serious defects and maximizing the chances of producing an example of excellence.

A master breeder needs several generations (a generation interval for horses is estimated to be 9–11 years) to create a pool of stock that contains the genetic elements that he or she considers to be important for the program vision. To learn to identify essential characteristics, a breeder needs to evaluate the horses and their pedigrees, not advertisements or pictures. When a breeder discovers those elements, he or she can make empirical judgments and is on an obvious path to making good breeding decisions.

The cult of the dominant sire

In some circles, the highest praise of a breeding stallion is that he is a dominant sire. Another widely encountered livestock breeding term for an elite sire is prepotency. The implication is that all his foals are stamped with his likeness, regardless of what mare is used. This concept would appear to contradict the advice to "start with a good mare". Those owners who strongly believe in the strengths and qualities of their breeding females would surely question the value of a so-called dominant sire who could seemingly obliterate valued characteristics that would be contributed by their mares.

A good understanding of genetics should allow a breeder to put the proper frame of reference to terms such as dominance and prepotency as applied to breeding horses. Some animals transmit certain characteristics at a higher frequency than is generally encountered with other breeding animals. Coat color is always the conspicuous example. Any stallion whose offspring always or nearly always match his color is popularly described as a dominant sire. To be exactly correct, for at least some of the effects being considered, the genetic interaction is not dominance but epistasis and homozygosity. A stallion could be homozygous for gray, leopard spotting, or tobiano, so that every foal, regardless of the color of the mare (with the possible exception of white), would have those traits. Homozygosity for color is not necessarily linked with the transmission of genes for good hoof structure, bone alignment in the front legs, shoulder angulation, or any other traits that may be desirable. Most conformation traits seem to be influenced by more than one gene. Some stallions may be exceptionally consistent sires of good conformational qualities, but it is unlikely that every foal will have these traits or that any stallion could be so characterized for more than a few traits.

The balanced view is that a battery of stallions is needed to meet the particular genetic requirements of each of the various mares in the breed. No one stallion can be the perfect sire for every mare's foal.

Using genetics to guide a breeding program

If assays for genes important for program goals are available, the probability of obtaining foals with selected traits from specific breeding pairs can be predicted. For many horse coat colors, offspring colors can be predicted, but conformation and performance traits are not well enough defined for predictive values to be assigned. So little is known about the genetics of desirable traits that it is premature to suggest that any general technique of structuring pedigrees consistently produces either better or worse stock.

The important lessons to learn from genetics for use in horse breeding decisions may seem nebulous to those looking for easy "how-to" information. Yet an appreciation of how genes are inherited, the number of genes involved in the makeup of a horse, their variability within a breed, and the inevitability of genetic trait reassortment with every individual in every generation will provide the critical foundation for sound breeding decisions.

With the current interest in genetics and the new technologies available for looking at genes at the molecular level, information about the inherited traits of horses is likely to increase significantly in the next decade. Horse owners can help with the process in several ways, including communication with granting agencies about specific problems of interest to them, providing money to fund the research, and providing information and tissue samples to funded research studies. Horse breeders are eager to have sound genetic information and diagnostic tests to guide their programs and, fortunately, the future looks very promising.

References

Cothran, E.G., MacCluer, J.W., Weitkamp, L.R., Pfenning, D.W. and Boyce, A.J. (1984) Inbreeding and reproductive performance in Standardbred horses. *Journal of Heredity* 75, 220–224.

Lush, J.L. (1945) *Animal Breeding Plans*. Iowa State University Press, Ames, Iowa.

MacCluer, J.W., Boyce, A.T., Dyke, B., Weitkamp, L.R., Pfenning, D.W. and Parsons, C.J. (1983) Inbreeding and pedigree structures in Standardbred horses. *Journal of Heredity* 74, 394–399.

van Vleck, L.D. (1990) Relationships and inbreeding. In: Evans, J.W., Borton, A., Hintz, H.F. and van Vleck, L.D. (eds) *The Horse*, 2nd edn. W.H. Freeman, New York, pp. 537–554.

16 Y Chromosomes, Mitochondria, Epigenetics, and Incomplete Penetrance

A recurring theme in this book is the equal genetic contribution from dam and sire. Gregor Mendel taught us that genes are discrete units inherited from both parents that may behave with a dominant, codominant or recessive modes of inheritance. Later, Thomas Hunt Morgan showed that these genes were present on chromosomes inherited from both parents and that gender was associated with the inheritance of chromosomes (Morgan, 1910). However, nature loves exceptions and scientists love discovering them. This chapter describes the small number of seeming exceptions to the Mendelian/Morganian modes of inheritance.

Y chromosomes, mitochondria, epigenetics and incomplete penetrance exhibit modes of inheritance that seemingly contradict the lessons from Gregor Mendel, yet this would be a misperception. The rules of Mendel apply to genes on autosomes. In the case of mitochondria and Y chromosomes, each has its own DNA which follows a unique pattern of inheritance. In the cases of genomic imprinting and incomplete penetrance, the genes may be inherited equally from sire or dam, but the expression of the genes is influenced by the gender of the parent (imprinting), or by the environment and chance events.

Y Chromosomes

Y chromosomes are only found in males and contain the genes responsible for initiating the development of male characteristics. The Y chromosome contains about 2% of the DNA found in a cell. In the absence of the Y chromosome, embryos develop female characteristics. We do not have an entire DNA sequence for the Y chromosome yet; it is difficult to sequence accurately because it is composed of large stretches of repetitive DNA that do not code for genes. Regions with repetitive sequences are prone to error during sequencing and assembly. But there is a small region (about 5% of the Y chromosome), called the pseudo-autosomal region (PAR) which contains genes and DNA similar to those found on the X chromosome, and actually pairs with the X chromosome during meiosis.

The number of genes in the PAR varies between species. We have the most information for the human Y chromosome, from which we know of at least 86 genes. Work is still underway at this writing to characterize the Y chromosome of horses, although at least 37 genes have been identified from the PAR region of the horse, with 20 of those appearing to be similar to those found on the X chromosome (and called degenerate X genes) (Paria *et al.*, 2011). The other 17 genes are unique to the Y chromosome; one of these is the *SRY* gene, which is responsible for the development of the testes.

Tail-male inheritance of the Y chromosome (paternal inheritance of Y chromosomes)

Because the Y chromosome only occurs in males, its inheritance follows the "tail-male" line in pedigrees (see Chapter 15). For example, over 95% of modern-day Thoroughbreds trace their ancestry to the Darley Arabian through the male side of the pedigree (tail-male). This means that 95% of the Thoroughbred stallions have the same Y chromosome as was found in the Darley Arabian. However, the DNA from the other chromosomes has been inherited from both parents, going right back to the foundation stock. Cunningham *et al.* (2001) determined that 158 founders contributed 81% of the DNA to modern-day Thoroughbred horses. The Darley Arabian contributed, on average, 6.5% of the DNA found in each of the modern-day Thoroughbreds. Ironically, the foundation sire the Goldophin Barb has the highest genetic contribution to Thoroughbred horses at 13.8%, though his Y chromosome is becoming lost to the breed as a consequence of his male descendants becoming uncommon.

DNA sequence variation of the Y chromosome among equids

However, the distinction of having the Y chromosome from the Darley Arabian or the Goldophin Barb may be of little consequence, as DNA sequences from 14,300 bases of the Y chromosome DNA of 52 horses from 15 breeds did not uncover any genetic variation among them (Lindgren *et al.*, 2004). Likewise, investigations of six Y chromosome microsatellites for 49 horses, and of 1–14 members of other equid species did not uncover variation among the horses but did uncover some genetic variation within the other species (Wallner *et al.*, 2004).

Later, scientists did uncover variation for one of the genetic markers among some horse breeds in southern China (Ling *et al.*, 2010). Interestingly, the Mongolian Wild horse (*Equus ferus przewalskii*) had two different haplotypes not found in the domestic horse (Wallner *et al.*, 2004). Together, these observations support several hypotheses: (i) variation in the Y chromosome of equids can exist among wild populations of equids: (ii) the very limited variation that appears to exist among domestic horses suggests that all domestic horses are descended from one or very few related stallions. Further to that hypothesis, this suggests that the stallions from one region were used in the first domestication event and that their male descendants were transported, worldwide, in concert with further domestication of the horse. When the Y chromosome is completely sequenced and assembled, we are likely to uncover yet more DNA variation, and the amount of variation found will allow us to better determine the role of stallions during the process of horse domestication.

Mitochondria

Mitochondria are small structures found within cells that carry out the important function of energy creation. The biochemistry of mitochondrial function falls outside the scope of this book, but basically, mitochondria are the sites where sugars are broken down in the manufacture of readily available energy for cells, namely adenosine triphosphate (ATP) molecules. For this reason, mitochondria are sometimes popularly referred to as the "powerhouse of the cell". Mitochondria are found in the cells of nearly all plants and animals. The number of mitochondria in a cell can vary depending on the energy needs of the cells. Cells in muscle, brain, and liver are very active and have many mitochondria.

Mitochondria have their own DNA. Within each mitochondrion, are 2–10 circular strands of DNA, each approximately 16,000 bases long and encoding 37 genes. Thirteen genes are for the generation of energy and 24 are for the enzymes necessary to translate the genes. The horse mitochondrion was sequenced and found to be similar to that of other species (Xu and Arnason, 1994). As described below, most of the genes responsible for the structure and function of horse mitochondria are actually found on chromosomes.

Are mitochondria descended from bacteria?

Mitochondrial DNA has properties more like bacterial DNA than chromosomal DNA. Like bacterial DNA, mitochondrial DNA is organized as a circular molecule and its genetic code also shows characteristics of bacterial DNA. One theory holds that the ancestors of mitochondria were once free-living bacteria that began living inside other cells. The bacteria inside the cells provided benefits to the host by producing prodigious amounts of ATP. Consequently, host cells with these bacteria were more successful in reproduction than cells without the mitochondria. As noted above, mitochondria are found in the cells of almost all plants and animals.

Mitochondrial DNA does not contain all the mitochondrial genes

Most of the genes that are responsible for the function of mitochondria are present on the chromosomes of the "host". Those genes are likely to have originated from the mitochondrial DNA when it was a component of a bacterium capable of independent existence. However, whenever DNA from the mitochondria broke free and became incorporated into chromosomes, the function of the mitochondria improved. By this process, most of the genes responsible for the structure and function of mitochondria are found on chromosomes. In the end, the mitochondria became an integral part of the cell and incapable of existence as an independent bacterial species.

Reproduction of mitochondria

Mitochondria reproduce by a method called binary fission, which the same method used by most bacteria. Unlike chromosomes, there is no pairing of DNA strands and no genetic recombination; simply, the DNA replicates and the mitochondrion divides into two equally functional parts. Furthermore, the reproduction of mitochondria is not coupled to cell division. Each cell can have hundreds or thousands of mitochondria, depending on the needs of the cell for energy.

Maternal inheritance of mitochondria

Mitochondrial DNA is passed from mothers to their offspring. When an egg is fertilized, the sperm contributes its chromosomal DNA only, and no mitochondria. The egg provides the maternal chromosomes and all the enzymes, structures, and materials necessary for a cell to function, including, of course, the mitochondria. As a consequence, all mitochondrial DNA comes from the dam. Regardless of the sex of the embryo, the mitochondrial DNA is maternal and the inheritance follows the "tail-female" line of a pedigree (see Chapter 15). As described above, the Y chromosome follows the tail-male line of a pedigree. This has consequences for the study of the origin and ancestry of horses.

Mitochondrial DNA has a higher mutation rate than chromosomal DNA

Mitochondrial DNA does not replicate as efficiently as chromosomal DNA. The DNA polymerase that replicates the mitochondrial DNA is not as effective at detecting and correcting errors as the DNA polymerase for chromosomes. Consequently, mutations occur in mitochondrial DNA at a much higher rate than that for chromosomal DNA. This is one reason why most of the genes migrated from the mitochondrial genome to the chromosomal genome. Genes that happened to break off from the mitochondrial DNA and became incorporated in chromosomal DNA were less likely to have deleterious mutations and the cells would enjoy more robust performance of the mitochondria.

Mitochondria and studies of breeds and evolution

Unlike the Y chromosome, the mitochondrial DNA of horses has been found to have lots of genetic variation. Mitochondrial DNA sequences have been used to investigate pedigree records (Bowling *et al.*, 2000; Hill *et al.*, 2002) and horse domestication (Vilà *et al.*, 2001; Jansen *et al.*, 2002). DNA sequencing from a short region, called the D-loop, was used to identify many mitochondrial DNA variants among horses. The DNA was from a region that did not have genes, so the mutations did not affect mitochondrial function. However, they were useful as a DNA clock to track the history of horses, including investigations of pedigree records and the history of domestication and breed development. The overall veracity of pedigree records following the female line was upheld, with a few historical errors identified, in studies of mitochondria from Arabian horses (Bowling *et al.*, 2000) and Thoroughbred horses (Hill *et al.*, 2002).

Mitochondrial DNA studies indicated that the domestication of horses involved many mares, presumably from diverse regions, in contrast the evidence indicating that few males contributed to the domestication events for horses (Vilà *et al.*, 2001; Jansen *et al.*, 2002). The studies suggest that the domestication of horses initially occurred in one region and was copied in other regions. As that occurred, stallions from the initial region were crossed with wild-caught mares from other areas. This would explain the limited variation that has been found for Y chromosome DNA, and the contrasting extensive variation of the mitochondrial DNA. This pattern of domestication is different from that for cattle, sheep, and pigs, in which it appears that domestication occurred in one region and then those domesticated animals were transported as breeding stock to other regions.

As the cost of DNA sequencing has decreased, it has become possible to compare horses for the entire mitochondrial genome sequence (Lippold *et al.*, 2011; Achilli *et al.*, 2012). Their observations have upheld the hypotheses constructed for domestication events and provided more information about the extent of variation. In addition, the studies have clearly demonstrated that most of the mitochondrial genotypes occur among all modern breeds and that all mitochondria DNA sequences could be derivative of an ancestral mitochondrion from 130 to 160 thousand years ago – the presumptive great-great-(and so on) – grandam of all horses.

Epigenetics

Epigenetics is a term used to denote heritable but potentially reversible changes in DNA. Unlike DNA mutations, the actual DNA sequence does not change in connection with epigenetic modification. Instead, enzymes add chemical groups to DNA bases or alter chromosomal proteins and make genes more or less accessible for expression. The changes are copied when the DNA is copied during cell division, but they can be readily reversed by the action of different enzymes. The changes are heritable in the sense that they are passed through meiotic cell division in the case of germinal cells (eggs and sperm) or through mitotic divisions in the cases of cells post fertilization.

The effects and mechanisms for epigenetics have not been extensively studied in horses; they are much better characterized for humans and mice (Feil and Fraga, 2012). Epigenetic modification appears to be a general feature of mammalian genetics, and we can anticipate that the lessons from humans, mice and other species will generally be applicable to horses. So far, we are aware of three general aspects of epigenetic changes: programming of tissues during development; environmentally induced changes; and associated genomic imprinting.

Epigenetic programming of tissues during development

The simplest example of epigenetic control of gene expression is the change which occurs in cells as they develop from fertilized eggs into fully differentiated tissues such as muscle, liver, kidney, and blood cells. The fertilized egg has the capacity to give rise to any cell type. Even though the muscle cell has all the genes that are found in the fertilized egg, it has been programmed in such a way that it cannot readily change into another type of cell. Changes in DNA methylation and in the proteins associated with chromosomes (histones) and chromatin structure help to regulate genes. The process of cell differentiation is one in which the number and type of genes that can be expressed is progressively diminished until the cell is "hard wired" for a specific cell type. The changes are unidirectional and cannot be reversed in nature, although in recent years scientists have discovered methods to reverse the changes when isolating and growing the cells in culture, thus giving rise to stem cells useful for cloning (Wilmut *et al.*, 1997).

Chapter 16

Environmentally induced epigenetic changes

Species are genetically adapted to their environment: it is, literally, "in their DNA", and determines such things as the types of foods they can eat and their levels of metabolism. However, in times of famine these genetic adaptations will not serve individuals well; selection for genes that increase appetite and lower metabolism will be more beneficial. But selecting for new genes will create more problems when the environmental change is short-term and original conditions return. For example, when the famine ends, the original genes will remain most adaptive. Evidence is mounting that epigenetic changes in gene expression provide a short-term, adaptive change that leaves the original genes intact. Specifically, studies of human populations and laboratory mice are uncovering evidence that these species adapt to short-term environmental changes by making epigenetic alterations to the genes of their off-spring (Hales and Barker, 2001).

For example, at the end of World War II, food supplies were severely restricted in Holland (the Netherlands), leading to widespread famine. Decades later, scientists noted that children born during and shortly following that period had adverse health problems throughout their lives; molecular genetic studies demonstrated the presence of markers for epigenetic change in affected individuals, but not in their siblings born after the famine (Heijmans *et al.*, 2008). The epigenetic changes affected genes that, under conditions of plentiful food and inactivity, are associated with the development of cardiovascular disease and metabolic syndrome (Tobi *et al.*, 2009).

Studies of laboratory mice provided experimental evidence for epigenetic responses to diet. The *Agouti* gene encodes a protein that binds a receptor regulating coat color when expressed in the skin and feeding behavior when expressed in the brain. Mice possessing the *Agouti* gene are typically obese with yellow colored fur. The *Agouti* gene was found to be under epigenetic control as a consequence of diet. The gene for this protein can be turned off by providing feed rich in methyl groups to mothers during pregnancy. Even though offspring had the *Agouti* gene, the high methyl group diet turned off expression of the protein, resulting in offspring that were small with brown fur; in the absence of high methyl groups in the feed, the gene was turned on and the offspring expressed the agouti protein, becoming obese and yellow colored (Morgan *et al.*, 1999; Waterland and Jirtle, 2003).

The main point here is that the DNA is not altered; however, changes in gene expression are passed on to subsequent generations. When exposure to environmental stimulus alters, then the epigenetic changes can be reversed. Studies have demonstrated epigenetic responses to cigarette smoke, toxins, diet, and exercise in humans and laboratory animals. Epigenetic response to environmental stimuli appear to be a general phenomenon which will certainly be applicable to horses and other livestock.

Genomic imprinting

Genomic imprinting describes the situation in which a gene is expressed based on the parent of origin. During egg development, certain genes are activated while others are turned off. Likewise, a different set of genes is activated and deactivated during sperm development. This parent-of-origin gene expression is regulated through the epigenetic mechanisms of DNA methylation and chromatin modification (McGrath and

Solter, 1984; Surani *et al.*, 1986). The result is that some genes are expressed only when they come from the dam and others are only expressed when they come from the sire. Only a small percentage of genes, less than 2% of the genome, exhibit this genomic imprinting.

Initial studies suggested that genomic imprinting of female gametes results in gene expression that promotes development of the placenta, but limits the demands of the fetus on her own health. Conversely, imprinting of male gametes tends to promote growth of the fetus even at the expense of the mother. There are exceptions that confound this hypothesis. Nevertheless, traits associated with early development and growth are attributable to exclusive expression from one parent or the other. For equids, this may explain the differences seen between mules and hinnies: mules are the products of jacks bred to mares while hinnies are the products of stallions bred to jennies. Studies of placental tissues from these crosses identified differences in gene expression that depended on the species of the sire or dam (Antczak *et al.*, 2012).

Genomic imprinting has been suggested to be responsible for the maternal grandam effect. Some Thoroughbred stallions have been identified as poor producers of racehorses but excellent grandsires through their filly offspring. The explanation might be that they have genes that are superior for racing performance, but which are only expressed when they are transmitted by a female (Antczak, Cornell University, Ithaca, New York, 2004, personal communication).

Incomplete Penetrance

This may seem an odd topic to include in this particular chapter because incomplete penetrance is often thought of as a mode of inheritance like dominance, codominance and recessiveness. "Incomplete penetrance" is usually defined as a situation where a gene or genotype is present but its corresponding/expected trait is not. In other words, the gene may or may not be expressed when present. This can happen in the following circumstances:

1. *Secondary genetic influences on gene expression.* The expression of a gene may be influenced by other genes. When present, a gene's expression may be blocked or decreased by other genetic influences. The condition associated with hyperkalemic periodic paralysis (HYPP) is a good example. Horses with HYPP have a gene defect that causes their skeletal muscles to act abnormally. The clinical expression of HYPP is highly variable among horses with the gene defect. Studies have shown that horses with less severe HYPP have a lower expression of the defective gene mRNA (Zhou *et al.*, 1994). We do not know why this difference exists among horses, but presumably is a consequence of action by yet other genes. In addition, muscle function is a complex trait and there are many genes and many pathways that influence muscle performance and might result in a decrease in the clinical signs.

2. *Genes expressed only upon exposure to pathogens.* Genes influence the clinical manifestation of infectious diseases. However, if horses do not encounter the pathogen, they will not have the opportunity to express the trait. When studying infectious diseases in natural populations, we do not know which horses have been exposed. The solution is to compare the frequency of candidate genes among affected horses with the frequency among other horses of the same breed or in the same family. An example of such work is the discovery of the association of sarcoid tumors in horses with the presence of the genes for certain equine lymphocyte antigens (ELAs) (Lazary *et al.*, 1985). Sarcoid tumors are benign growths of skin cells resulting from infection with papilloma viruses. Lazary *et al.* (1985) determined that all affected offspring from stallions inherited the genes for lymphocyte antigens from only one of the stallions' two chromosomes. Some unaffected horses also had that lymphocyte antigen though there was no way of knowing whether or not they had had the same exposure to the papilloma virus.

3. *Gene expression dependent upon management.* The expression of a gene may be dependent upon the management of a horse. As noted above and in Chapter 12, HYPP is a hereditary disease of horses. If horses with the gene for HYPP are maintained on a low potassium diet without stress, the condition may not be apparent (Reynolds *et al.*, 1998). Likewise, other disease genes or performance characteristics may depend upon a particular management style or nutrition.

4. *Random aspects of gene expression.* Every cell in the body of a tobiano patterned horse has the gene that causes depigmentation. Why some cells are depigmented and others are not is not known.

The genes that we understand best of all are those which are always expressed when present in the appropriate genotype (homozygous or heterozygous). They are easy and unambiguous to find, and include many of the disease genes and coat color pattern genes described in earlier chapters. For example, all horses with two copies of the gene for severe combined immunodeficiency (SCID, see Chapter 12) fail to develop an effective immune system and die during the first 6 months from opportunistic infections. No exceptions have been seen.

As another example, all horses with the gray hair gene become gray. In this case too, no exceptions have been seen, although the age of onset for graying may vary considerably and we might consider this aspect of gene expression as being incompletely penetrant. Further, even though we tend to regard genes as having dominant or recessive characteristics, many of the traits that interest us and many of the diseases that bedevil us probably exhibit some aspect of incomplete penetrance.

References

Achilli, A. *et al.* (2012) Mitochondrial genomes from modern horses reveal the major haplogroups that underwent domestication. *Proceedings of the National Academy of Sciences of the United States of America* 109, 2449–2454.

Antczak, D.F., Xu, W., Miller, D. and Clark, A.G. (2012) Imprinted genes in placenta and fetus of horse × donkey hybrids. In: *Proceedings of Plant and Animal Genome XIX Conference, January 15–19, 2011, Town and Country Convention Center, San Diego, CA,* W018: Animal Epigenetics, Abstract. Available at: http://www.intlpag.org/2013/index.php/archives/pg-i-to-pag-xix-archives (accessed 24 January 2013).

Bowling, A.T., Del Valle, A. and Bowling, M. (2000) A pedigree-based study of mitochondrial D-loop DNA sequence variation among Arabian horses. *Animal Genetics* 31, 1–7.

Cunningham, E.P., Dooley, J.J., Splan, R.K. and Bradley, D.G. (2001) Microsatellite diversity, pedigree relatedness and the contributions of founder lineages to Thoroughbred horses. *Animal Genetics* 32, 360–364.

Feil, R. and Fraga, M.F. (2012) Epigenetics and the environment: emerging patterns and implications. *Nature Reviews Genetics* 13, 97–109.

Hales, C.N. and Barker, D.J. (2001) The thrifty phenotype hypothesis. *British Medical Bulletin* 60, 5–20.

Heijmans, B.T., Tobi, E.W., Stein, A.D., Putter, H., Blauw, G.J., Susser, E.S., Slagboom, P.E. and Lumey, L.H. (2008) Persistent epigenetic differences associated with prenatal exposure to famine in humans. *Proceedings of the National Academy of Sciences of the United States of America* 105, 17046–17049.

Hill, E.W., Bradley, D.G., Al-Barody, M., Ertugrul, O., Splan, R.K., Zakharov, I. and Cunningham, E.P. (2002) History and integrity of Thoroughbred dam lines revealed in equine mtDNA variation. *Animal Genetics* 33, 287–294.

Jansen, T., Forster, P., Levine, M.A., Oelke, H., Hurles, M., Renfrew, C., Weber, J. and Olek, K. (2002) Mitochondrial DNA and the origins of the domestic horse. *Proceedings of the National Academy of Sciences of the United States of America* 99, 10905–10910.

Lazary, S., Gerber, H., Glatt, P.A. and Straub, R. (1985) Equine leucocyte antigens in sarcoid-affected horses. *Equine Veterinary Journal* 17, 283–286.

Lindgren, G., Backström, N., Swinburne, J., Hellborg, L., Einarsson, A., Sandberg, K., Cothran, G., Vilà, C., Binns, M. and Ellegren, H. (2004) Limited number of patrilines in horse domestication. *Nature Genetics* 36, 335–336.

Ling, Y., Ma, Y., Guan, W., Cheng, Y., Wang, Y., Han, J., Jin, D., Mang, L and Mahmut, H. (2010) Identification of Y chromosome genetic variations in Chinese indigenous horse breeds. *Journal of Heredity* 10, 639–643.

Lippold, S., Knapp, M., Kuznetsova, T., Leonard, J.A., Benecke, N., Ludwig, A., Rasmussen, M., Cooper, A., Weinstock, J., Willerslev, E., Shapiro, B. and Hofreiter, M. (2011) Discovery of lost diversity of paternal horse lineages using ancient DNA. *Nature Communications* 2, 450.

McGrath, J. and Solter, D. (1984) Inability of mouse blastomere nuclei transferred to enucleated zygotes to support development in vitro. *Science* 226, 1317–1319.

Morgan, H.D., Sutherland, H.G., Martin, D.I. and Whitelaw, E. (1999) Epigenetic inheritance at the agouti locus in the mouse. *Nature Genetics* 23, 314–318.

Morgan, T.H. (1910) Sex limited inheritance in *Drosophila*. *Science* 32, 120–122.

Paria, N., Raudsepp, T., Pearks Wilkerson, A.J., O'Brien, P.C., Ferguson-Smith, M.A., Love, C.C., Arnold, C., Rakestraw, P., Murphy, W.J. and Chowdhary, B.P. (2011) A gene catalogue of the euchromatic male-specific region of the horse Y chromosome: comparison with human and other mammals. *PLoS One* 6(7): e21374, doi: 10.1371/journal.pone.0021374.

Reynolds, J.A., Potter, G.D., Greene, L.W., Wu, G., Carter, K., Martin, M.T., Peterson, T.V., Murra, Y., Gerzik, M., Moss, G. and Erkert, R.S. (1998) Genetic–diet interactions in the hyperkalemic periodic paralysis syndrome in Quarter Horses fed varying amounts of potassium: I. Potassium and sodium balance, packed cell volume and plasma potassium, and sodium concentrations. *Journal of Equine Veterinary Science* 18, 591–600.

Surani, M.A., Barton, S.C. and Norris, M.L. (1986) Nuclear transplantation in the mouse: heritable differences between parental genomes after activation of the embryonic genome. *Cell* 45, 127–136.

Tobi, E.W., Lumey, L.H., Talens, R.P., Kremer, D., Putter, H., Stein, A.D., Slagboom, P.E. and Heijmans, B.T. (2009) DNA methylation differences after exposure to prenatal famine are common and timing- and sex-specific. *Human Molecular Genetics* 18, 4046–4053.

Vilà, C., Leonard, J.A., Gotherstrom, A., Marklund, S., Sandberg, K., Liden, K., Wayne, R.K. and Ellegren, H. (2001) Widespread origins of domestic horse lineages. *Science* 291, 474–477.

Wallner, B., Piumi, F., Brem, G., Müller, M. and Achmann, R. (2004) Isolation of Y chromosome-specific microsatellites in the horse and cross-species amplification in the genus *Equus*. *Journal of Heredity* 95, 158–164.

Waterland, R.A. and Jirtle, R.L. (2003) Transposable elements: targets for early nutritional effects on epigenetic gene regulation. *Molecular and Cellular Biology* 23, 5293–5300.

Wilmut, I., Schnieke, A.E., McWhir, J., Kind, A.J. and Campbell, K.H. (1997) Viable offspring derived from fetal and adult mammalian cells. *Nature* 385, 810–813.

Xu, X. and Arnason, U. (1994) The complete mitochondrial DNA sequence of the horse, *Equus caballus*: extensive heteroplasmy of the control region. *Gene* 148, 357–362.

Zhou, J., Spier, S.J., Beech, J. and Hoffman, E.P. (1994) Pathophysiology of sodium channelopathies: correlation of normal/mutant mRNA ratios with clinical phenotype in dominantly inherited periodic paralysis. *Human Molecular Genetics* 3, 1599–1603.

17 Genetic Nature of Breeds

Historically, horse breeds were defined by geography (e.g. Arabian, Shire, Exmoor), but in the present day sense, a breed is defined by breeder societies as a population of related horses with specific characteristics. Breeds may be distinctive for innate abilities such as gait, power, speed, or endurance. The appearance and behavior of individual horses may even make it possible distinguish between horse breeds. At the same time, horses of different breeds can also appear very similar if they shared ancestry and have common uses.

Breed Registries and Purebred Horses

The goal for a breed registry is to improve its breed. Typically, registries keep pedigree records (the stud book) and establish rules for registration. They may also establish rules for the comparison or competition of their horses. When a horse is descended from parents that belong to a registry, it is considered to be purebred.

One of the most famous pedigree records is the *General Stud Book*, begun in 1793 by the Thoroughbred horse registry in the UK (which is historically known as The Jockey Club or Weatherbys). Thoroughbred racing has become popular worldwide and additional registries exist for Thoroughbred horses in countries wherever Thoroughbred racing occurs. All Thoroughbred racehorse registries cooperate under the aegis of an organization called the International Stud Book Committee (ISBC). Similar arrangements exist for other breeds, with registries being local, national, or international in character.

Fundamentally, a registry is composed of individuals who desire to produce horses with specific characteristics and lay out criteria for the inclusion of horses. To start with, the criteria may be a set of phenotypic characters, including color or a time standard for racing or the ability to perform a particular gait. The traits are heritable and pedigrees records are maintained. When registry owners agree that no genetic improvement will occur by the addition of horses from outside the pedigree, they may "close the book". A registry with a "closed book" requires that a registered horse must also have registered parents. Horses from registries with closed books are often described as "purebred" because they, as well as both parents, were registered.

Notice that "purebred" is an administrative and cultural definition, not a genetic one. Purebred horses are not genetically identical. Indeed, if they were, then blood typing or DNA testing would not be able to uniquely identify horses and parentage testing would be moot. The genetic foundation of breeds has been quite diverse and the variation among horses a source of enjoyment for breeders. As described in Chapter 3, we know that there are 2.43 billion DNA bp and over 20,000 genes, which are regulated in a complex fashion and result in literally countless combinations and genuinely unique characters.

Genetic variation within a breed

Some physical traits are characteristic of breeds. The Arabian horse is renowned for its concave (dish) face and a slight bulge between the eyes called the jibbah (Plate 20). But not all Arabian horses have these characteristics. There are physiognomic traits that are hereditary, variable and more common in one breed (for example, Arabians) than in others. If we came upon a horse without a dish face and jibbah, we might have more difficulty ascertaining whether or not it was an Arabian horse. We would look at the tail carriage, nostril flare, shape of the throatlatch, and other characteristics to refine our decision. However, if the horse under examination was part of a herd in which 70% of the horses exhibited these distinctive traits, we would be confident identifying the horse as part of the Arabian breed. Conversely, the existence of a jibbah in a random horse would not necessarily be proof that the horse was an Arabian because the characteristic can occur in other horse breeds.

In the 1950s and 1960s, scientists began discovering genetic variation for blood group and biochemical markers in horses. The genes included were those of eight blood group systems and many biochemical systems, such as transferrin, hemoglobin, albumin, serum esterase, proteases, and a variety of enzymes found in serum and red blood cells (Sandberg and Cothran, 2000). Lots of variation was found and the tests were useful for parentage testing. No genetic markers were ever found to be unique to a particular breed or even to a particular type of horse, although most genes did exhibit differences in their distribution among breeds. For example, the alleles A and B for the two common types of albumin (albumin A – ALB-A; and albumin B – ALB-B), occur among horses of all breeds, but studies have shown that the frequency of those alleles varies between breeds. Some breeds have a higher frequency of A than B, while others have a higher frequency of B than A. These frequency differences were stable from farm to farm as long as horses belonged to a particular breed. The conclusions from these studies were that: (i) all horse populations are closely related and share the same genes and alleles; and (ii) the development of breeds has resulted in gene frequency differences between the populations. It is a bit like baking: pasta, bread, cakes and biscuits have the same ingredient but in different proportions. The beginning point for comparing horse breeds is to identify the differences in gene frequencies between breeds.

Calculating Gene Frequencies for Dominant or Codominant Alleles

We do not know which genes or even the number of genes that determine whether a horse's nose is concave, flat or Roman shaped. But we can identify other genes and determine gene frequencies. The gene for albumin mentioned above is a good example. Albumin is a protein that is found abundantly in the blood. Genetic tests have long existed to characterize the albumin alleles into their two types, A and B. Each horse gets one set of chromosomes from each of its two parents so it will have two copies of the albumin gene (*ALB*). Therefore, the possible albumin genotypes for a horse are *AA*, *AB* and *BB*, corresponding to phenotypes ALB-A, ALB-AB and ALB-B. Because the gene for albumin has a dominant (or codominant) mode of expression, we can determine the gene frequency for each of the albumin alleles by simple counting, as shown in the example below.

In a sample of 9848 Paso Finos, there were 1703 horses of phenotype ALB-A (genotype *AA*), 4799 of phenotype ALB-AB (genotype *AB*), and 3346 of phenotype ALB-B (genotype *BB*) (Bowling, 1996). So:

- the total number of alleles is 19,696 (twice the number of horses);
- the number of *A* alleles is (2 × 1703) + 4799 = 8205;
- the number of *B* alleles is (2 × 3346) + 4799 = 11,491;
- the frequency of *A* is 8025/19,696 = 0.42; and
- the frequency of *B* is 11,491/19,696 = 0.58.

(Try calculating allelic frequencies for albumin in another breed: among 31,179 Arabians were 6114 horses of type ALB-A, 14,915 of type ALB-AB and 10,690 of type ALB-B. Check your calculations by comparing your answers with the albumin allele frequencies given for Arabian horses in Table 17.1.)

From Table 17.1, you can see that both alleles for albumin are found in all breeds of horses. The presence of either or both alleles in an individual horse tells us nothing about the breed of the horse. However, if we were to find a pasture with 100 horses of the same breed, type them for albumin, and find a frequency for the *B* allele of 0.45, we would reject the suggestion that the horses were Lippizaners, Miniature Horses or Thoroughbreds: the frequency of the *B* allele would be too high. Of course, we would also draw this conclusion from other observations, but the main point is that the gene frequencies for albumin alleles gives us evidence for and against the breed membership for a *herd* of horses. As we test a larger number of genes, our evidence becomes stronger, although we have never found a gene that is characteristic of a particular breed. While horses of all breeds can have albumin allele *A* and albumin allele *B*, the

Table 17.1. Frequencies of the albumin gene (*ALB*) alleles (*A* and *B*) among 13 horse breeds as determined by counting.

Breed	Frequency of *A*	Frequency of *B*
Andalusian	0.59	0.41
Arabian	0.43	0.57
Belgian	0.35	0.65
Icelandic	0.43	0.57
Lippizaner	0.08	0.92
Miniature	0.27	0.73
Norwegian Fjord	0.34	0.66
Paso Fino	0.42	0.58
Quarter Horse	0.28	0.72
Shire	0.45	0.55
Standardbred	0.59	0.41
Tennessee Walking horse	0.44	0.56
Thoroughbred	0.17	0.83

frequency of the alleles in a population of horses provides a small piece of evidence for the breed of origin.

The Hardy–Weinberg equation (HWE)

Gene frequencies are very useful for comparing breeds, but genes occur in pairs, one from the sire and one from the dam. If we want to know how many homozygotes and heterozygotes will occur, we use the Hardy–Weinberg equation (HWE). The main elements of the HWE are can be shown using the the Punnett square that was described in Chapter 2.

The frequency of sperm with A alleles is 0.50 and the frequency of sperm with the B allele is also 0.50. The frequencies are the same (0.50) for eggs with A or B alleles. The chances of an egg with the A allele being fertilized by a sperm with an A allele is $0.50 \times 0.50 = 0.25$, or a 25% chance of a homozygote for A. The same is true for homozygotes for B. For heterozygotes (AB), there are two ways to produce this genotype: an egg with B fertilized by a sperm with A (25%), or an egg with A fertilized by a sperm with B (25%) for a total of 50% AB. The ratio is 1:2:1.

Although Table 17.2 represents the mating of two horses, we can use the same approach to study the expected distribution of homozygotes and heterozygotes in populations. Table 17.3 shows a Punnett square that uses the frequencies for the A and B alleles in the Thoroughbred horse populations (Table 17.1) in place of the proportion of A and B possessing eggs and sperm in heterozygotes (Table 17.2). In this case, Table 17.3 demonstrates that 3% of the Thoroughbreds should be homozygotes for A, 69% homozygotes for B, and 28% (14% + 14%) heterozygotes for AB. In this example, we assumed that the allele frequencies were the same for stallions and mares. Notice that the gene frequency for A is 0.17 (17% of all albumin genes) but that only 3% of the offspring are homozygous for A. If this were the gene for a recessive disease trait, such as severe combined immunodeficiency (SCID), you can see how a relatively high gene frequency can occur while the number of affected individuals remains small. Furthermore, because heterozygotes are silent carriers of recessive genes, a gene frequency of 17% corresponds to having 28% carriers. It would take a long time to get rid of a recessive disease gene without identifying all carriers for negative selection.

Tables like 17.2 and 17.3 are useful for explaining the relationships among genes but are awkward for calculations. The HWE concisely expresses the relationships from the tables and is easily modified for calculating more complicated genetic relationships, including genetic systems with more than two alleles, multiple loci, and

Table 17.2. Punnett square showing the expectations for foals from the mating of two parents heterozygous for the albumin gene (*ALB*) alleles *A* and *B* (*AB* × *AB*).

Contribution from mare	Contribution from stallion	
	A (50%)	B (50%)
A (50%)	AA (25%)	AB (25%)
B (50%)	AB (25%)	BB (25%)

Table 17.3. Punnett square showing the frequencies of the different genotypic classes for albumin among Thoroughbred horses.

Contribution from mare	Contribution from stallion	
	Frequency of A (0.17 = 17%)	Frequency of B (0.83 = 83%)
Frequency of A (0.17 = 17%)	AA (0.17 × 0.17 = 0.03 = 3%)	AB (0.17 × 0.83 = 0.14 = 14%)
Frequency of B (0.83 = 83%)	AB (0.17 × 0.83 = 0.14 = 14%)	BB (0.83 × 0.83 = 0.69 = 69%)

the inclusion of genetic selection, genetic drift, and mutation. When this is done, the HWE takes the following basic form:

$$1 = p^2 + 2pq + q^2$$

where 1 is the sum of all the frequencies for all homozygotes and heterozygotes, p is the frequency of one allele and q is the frequency of the other allele. These elements are clearly represented in the Punnett square format. In the main body of the table, the p^2 represents the value in the upper left corner (frequency of homozygotes for one allele), the q^2 represents the value in the lower left corner (frequency of homozygotes for the second allele); and the $2pq$ represents the sum of the values in the upper right and lower left (all the heterozygotes). The modifications are described in many standard genetics textbooks on population genetics.

Calculating gene frequencies for recessive alleles

Sometimes we want to know about recessive alleles within a breed. We cannot simply count the number of alleles of each type. When an allele is recessive, it is not expressed and carriers are indistinguishable from non-carriers. However, we can use part of the HWE to determine the gene frequency of the recessive gene. There is no question but that the horses exhibiting the recessive trait are homozygous for that allele. The horses exhibiting the recessive trait will occur in a breed at a frequency of p^2, which leads to the following equation:

$$p = \sqrt{\frac{\text{No. horses with recessive trait}}{\text{No. horses examined}}}$$

This formula is useful for calculating the frequency of recessive alleles such as chestnut coat color, non-gray coat color, and the recessive disease alleles for SCID, lavender foal syndrome (LFS), junctional epidermolysis bullosa (JEB) and foal immunodeficiency syndrome (FIS). We can carry this calculation one step further and determine the carrier rate for the recessive gene. The carrier rate for recessive alleles is $2pq$, where q is the frequency of the dominant allele and $q = (1 - p)$.

Genetic Diversity, Genetic Drift, and Selection

The process of breed formation is a process of reducing genetic diversity in a population. Breeders want to increase alleles that contribute to the desired phenotype and eliminate alleles that adversely affect the horse. Two processes predominate: genetic drift and selection.

Genetic drift

With respect to the 2.43 billion DNA bp and 20,000-plus genes that make up the horse genome, the amount of variation within a breed is determined by the number and variety of horses that make up that breed. As long as the registry maintains an open book, new gene variants may be introduced into the population with new horses. Once the book is closed, the sum total of genes is precisely determined by the founders of the breed. It is true that mutation can create new genetic variants in such a closed population, but this is an uncommon event. From a pragmatic viewpoint, the genetic universe of a breed is determined by the number of horses included (founders) before the book is closed.

Events unrelated to selection can have an impact on the presence of an allele. One of these is called genetic drift. Alleles that are rare in the population are at great risk of being lost. If a genetic variant occurs in only one individual, or in only a few individuals, and by chance that allele is not passed on to the next generation, then the allele will no longer exist in that breed. Genetic diversity will decrease. Conservation biologists are concerned about loss of genetic diversity because some genes may provide the capacity to resist epidemic disease or to otherwise increase fitness in a changing environment. We cannot know the value of each and every gene, so breeders are encouraged to value genetic diversity in breeding programs.

In some instances, genetic drift can actually increase the frequency of an allele. One example comes from the D blood group system of horses. Before the use of DNA typing, blood typing was used to conduct parentage testing in horses (reviewed in Sandberg and Cothran, 2000). The D blood group system was one of the most useful systems as it contains more than 20 alleles. The allele for the blood group factor Dcf was very rare among horses, only being seen in few breeds other than American Standardbreds. The frequency of the *Dcf* allele was less than 0.005 before 1965 (Bailey, unpublished data). However, in 1960, an American Standardbred pacer colt inherited this allele from his dam. He went on to become a very successful racehorse and later a very popular breeding sire. By 1986, the frequency of the Dcf blood group among pacers was 0.05, a greater than 100-fold increase since 1965 (Cothran *et al.*, 1987). This blood group factor has no known impact on racing performance, fertility, or disease resistance that would explain its selection. The most likely explanation for the increased frequency is coincidence with the popularity of this stallion as a sire. Sometimes, this type of gene frequency change is referred to as "founder effect" as the drift is an inadvertent aspect of selection.

Selection

Selection causes changes in gene frequencies as a result of choices made by breeders to use particular animals as breeding stock. These choices should lead to the gain of genes that make the horse more desirable and the loss of genes that do not improve the phenotype. Until recently, we have not been able to identify any performance genes at the molecular level, so direct selection for genes has not occurred. Consequently, we can only speculate that differences in gene frequency for certain genes are related to performance. In a few years, we may have direct evidence about the role of genes and performance for some traits.

The gene for myostatin (*MSTN*) is one that may have an impact on horse racing performance. This gene was initially described for Thoroughbred racehorses and has two variants, which are described in some reports as "C" for the "sprint allele" and "T" for the "endurance allele" (Binns *et al.*, 2010; Hill *et al.*, 2010; Tozaki *et al.*, 2010). The endurance allele, *T*, has a high frequency among Arabian horses ($T = 0.92$; $C = 0.08$) that have been selected for endurance while the allele associated with speed (*C*) has a high frequency among Quarter Horses ($T = 0.10$; $C = 0.90$) that have been selected for sprinting distances of 400 m or less (Bower *et al.*, 2012). We cannot know for certain, but it is likely that selection for speed has increased the sprinting allele for Quarter Horses, while selection for stamina has led to the endurance allele being most common among Arabian horses.

Genetic Relationships Among Breeds

As described above, geneticists typically use gene frequencies to compare breeds. One of the first comprehensive comparisons of gene frequencies in horse breeds was reported using 20 blood group and biochemical markers for seven horse breeds that are common in the USA (Bowling and Clark, 1985). The work showed distinctive differences in gene frequencies between breeds as well as distinctive differences in the extent of genetic variation. Later, DNA markers became available and have been used widely to compare horses. These studies have benefited greatly from the increased use of parentage testing by horse breed registries around the world and adoption of a common set of microsatellite DNA markers for routine testing. Figure 17.1 shows a genetic tree representing the relationship among 2583 horses of 40 horse breeds, plus the miniature donkey, tested with 15 microsatellite DNA markers (Conant *et al.*, 2012). The authors noted three major divisions among breeds: "In this tree, the main clades are pony and draft horses, South American breeds of Iberian origin, and Old World and North American breeds". The value of these studies is to show the extent to which horse breeds share genetic markers as a reflection of their natural history, domestication, and selection.

The development of genetic markers based on SNPs (see Chapter 3) provides greater resolution for investigations of relationships among horse breeds. Figure 17.2 illustrates the results of analyses of genetic distance in 38 horse populations using 6028 SNP markers (Petersen *et al.*, 2013). Many of the breeds represented in Fig. 17.2 also appear in Fig. 17.1. Although the formats of the two figures are different, the groupings remain fundamentally the same.

Genetic markers for identification of breeds

A common question has been: "Can we tell the breed of a horse by its genetic markers?" We have seen that we can distinguish among horse breeds by studying gene frequencies in groups of horses. What about a single horse? What power do we have to determine its breed?

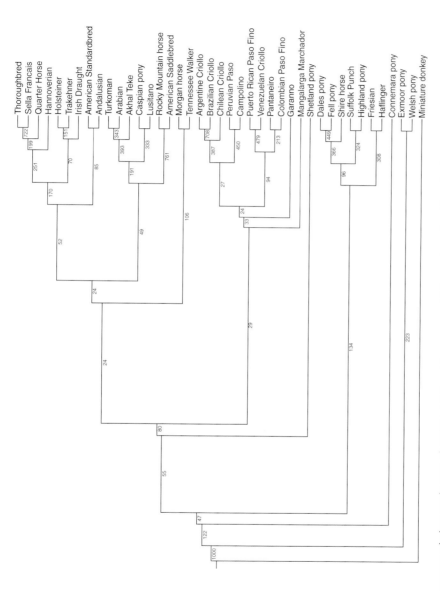

Fig. 17.1. Consensus phylogenetic tree showing relationships among 40 horse breeds with a donkey out-group based on testing with 15 microsatellite DNA markers. Restricted maximum likelihood (RML) trees based on chord distance were generated from 1000 bootstrapped allele frequency data sets, and majority-rule consensus trees created from the RML trees. The figures on the branches indicate bootstrap values. Reprinted with permission from Conant *et al.* (2012).

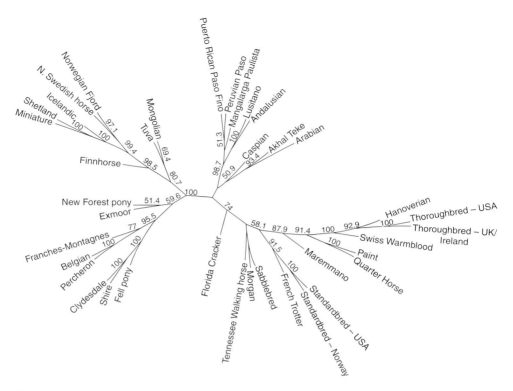

Fig. 17.2. Majority rule, neighbor join tree created from 6028 SNP markers using Nei's genetic distance and allele frequencies within each population. The percentage bootstrap support indicated on all branches was calculated from 1000 replicates. Reprinted with permission from Petersen *et al.* (2013).

In one example from above, the frequency of the *Dcf* allele for a rare blood group factor in the D blood group system was amplified in the American Standardbred pacing horse population by the use of a popular stallion. The allele is rare among all horse breeds and when a horse has one, it is likely to be a Standardbred pacer. However, the allele has been seen in other breeds in other parts of the world (anecdotal reports to author at ISAG (International Society of Animal Genetics) workshops). Therefore, the presence of *Dcf* is not proof, by itself, that a horse is an American Standardbred pacer. Conversely, the allele remains at a low frequency, and its absence does not mean that the horse is not an American Standardbred pacer. Clearly, we need to use more markers.

Bjørnstad and Røed (2001) conducted a study of 306 horses from eight horse breeds commonly found in Norway using 26 microsatellite DNA markers. The analysis they undertook was similar to the one illustrated in Fig. 17.1; it investigated the relationship among breeds and created a genetic tree. The authors then investigated the alleles found in each horse to see whether the combination of alleles would logically lead to a correct breed assignment based on the relative frequency among all the breeds tested. Of 306 horses in their study, correct assignments were made for 276. Mis-assignments were found only for horses from closely related breeds – specifically, breeds that had recently diverged. These results are exciting and suggest some efficacy for this approach.

Chapter 17

We can also see that genetic tests used to identify the breed of a single horse are limited by three factors: (i) the number of markers tested; (ii) the number of horses tested for comparison; and (iii) the number of breeds tested as reference populations. The more markers tested and the more reference animals for comparison, the more accurate the answer. Furthermore, the nature of the question means that assignments will only be made to breeds that have been identified beforehand. The testing of crossbred horses poses special problems for this statistical approach.

Genetic marker testing to investigate ancestry has become available for human genealogists wishing to investigate their own ancestry using human DNA markers. The results do not constitute proof for a pedigree, though the information may suggest a connection that would be personally gratifying. When the ancestors of a particular family line cannot be identified and Irish ancestry is suspected, then identifying genetic markers that are common among Irish populations may alleviate some disappointment at not finding civic or church records to build the genealogical record. This application of genetics has come to be called, "recreational genetics".

Finally, breeds are human inventions using pedigrees as proxies for genetics. It seems ironic then that we now use genetics as a proxy for pedigrees.

References

Binns, M.M., Boehler, D.A. and Lambert, D.H. (2010) Identification of the myostatin locus (*MSTN*) as having a major effect on optimum racing distance in the Thoroughbred horse in the USA. *Animal Genetics* 41 (Supplement 2),154–158.

Bjørnstad, G. and Røed, K.H. (2001) Breed demarcation and potential for breed allocation of horses assessed by microsatellite markers. *Animal Genetics* 32, 59–65.

Bower, M.A. *et al.* (2012) The genetic origin and history of speed in the Thoroughbred racehorse. *Nature Communications* 24, 643, doi:10.1038/ncomms1644.

Bowling, A.T. (1996) *Horse Genetics.* CAB International, Wallingford, UK, pp. 146–147.

Bowling, A.T. and Clark, R.S. (1985) Blood group and protein polymorphism gene frequencies for seven breeds of horses in the United States. *Biochemical Genetics* 16, 93–108.

Conant, E.K., Juras, R. and Cothran, E.G. (2012) A microsatellite analysis of five Colonial Spanish horse populations of the southeastern United States. *Animal Genetics* 43, 53–62.

Cothran, E.G., MacCluer, J.W., Weitkamp, L.R. and Bailey, E. (1987) Genetic differentiation associated with gait within American Standardbred horses. *Animal Genetics* 18, 285–296.

Hill, E.W., McGivney, B.A., Gu, J., Whiston, R. and MacHugh, D.E. (2010) A genome-wide SNP-association study confirms a sequence variant (g.66493737C>T) in the equine myostatin (*MSTN*) gene as the most powerful predictor of optimum racing distance for Thoroughbred racehorses. *BMC Genomics* 11: 552, doi:10.1186/1471-2164-11-552.

Petersen, J.L. *et al.* (2013) Genetic diversity in the modern horse illustrated from genome-wide SNP data. *PLOS One* (in press).

Sandberg, K. and Cothran, E.G. (2000) Biochemical genetics and blood groups. In: Bowling, A.T. and Ruvinsky, A. (eds) *The Genetics of the Horse.* CAB International, Wallingford, pp. 85–108.

Tozaki, T., Miyake, T., Kakoi, H., Gawahara, H., Sugita, S., Hasegawa, T., Ishida, N., Hirota, K. and Nakano, Y. (2010) A genome-wide association study for racing performances in Thoroughbreds clarifies a candidate region near the *MSTN* gene. *Animal Genetics* 41 (Supplement 2), 28–35.

18 *Equus*

In the Linnaean system of organizing the living world, equids are classified as follows:

Kingdom: Animal
Phylum: Vertebrate
Class: Mammalia
Order: Perissodactyla
Family: Equidae
Genus: *Equus*

The Perissodactyla are herbivorous, hoofed mammals with an odd toe number. The closest living relatives to the Equidae are the other perissodactyls – the rhinoceros (Fig. 18.1), and the tapir (Fig. 18.2). For a more detailed discussion of the family, consult Groves and Ryder (2000). The only extant members of the Equidae family are also members of the genus *Equus*. They are generally regarded as belonging to four major groups: the horses (domestic horses and Przewalski's horse), the donkeys (the domestic donkey and Somali wild ass), the Asiatic wild asses (hemiones and kiangs), and the zebras (*E. quagga*, *E. zebra*, *E. grevyi*). Each species has the same general morphology and size as the domestic horse, but only the horse and donkey have been amenable to domestication. Despite their similar appearances, each species evolved separately and each is uniquely adapted to different regions of the world. Consequently, they exhibit unique behaviors, unique physical characteristics, and unique genetic attributes.

Classification and Differences Among Equids

Species classification and population standings

The classification of the Equidae is based on the Linnaean system as recommended through agencies of the nongovernmental organization the International Union for Conservation of Nature (IUCN). IUCN is devoted to global environmental science and the maintenance of biological diversity. When defining a biological species, scientists take into account physical characteristics and geographical distribution, as well as biological abilities to reproduce, behavioral barriers to reproduction, and genetic measures of evolutionary distance between populations. In former times, the separation of two populations by a mountain range may have been sufficient for the populations to have accumulated genetic, physical, and behavioral differences that merited their consideration as a discrete and unique population. In modern times, with pressure from growing human populations and

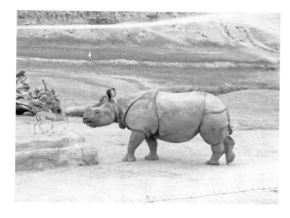

Fig. 18.1. Indian rhinoceros.

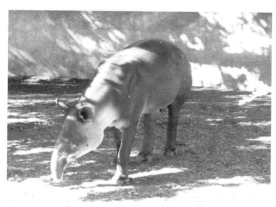

Fig. 18.2. Central American tapir.

mechanized travel, many small populations of animals have been pushed together, forcing the hybridization of groups of animals that had diverged significantly. As a result, precisely defining species and their characteristics can be challenging. Nevertheless, geneticists have been resourceful in applying a wide variety of techniques, including DNA sequencing, to discover and characterize the diverse species.

Chromosomal differences among the Equidae species

Chromosomal morphology and numbers in the living members of the genus *Equus* present a heterogeneous picture. As an illustration of this diversity, the chromosome numbers found for the species (and some subspecies) of the four major groups noted above are shown in Table 18.1. The scientific name of the species is given in the far left column, followed in subsequent columns by common names and the number of chromosomes reported for each species. The practice is to type the genus and species name in full the first time it is used, and then simply abbreviate it with the first letter(s) thereafter. So *Equus ferus caballus* becomes *E. f. caballus*.

Each species of *Equus* has a different numbers of chromosomes. This is not always the case among mammalian families. For example, almost all members of the cat family have 38 chromosomes, from lions to the domestic house cat. For the genus *Equus*, the chromosome number is characteristic of most species.

The chromosomes of domestic horses and donkeys are well known from clinical karyotyping studies, as well as genome mapping studies, and excellent idiograms exist that depict the number and structure of the chromosomes (Bowling *et al.*, 1997; Raudsepp *et al.*, 2000; Di Meo *et al.*, 2009). However, relatively fewer karyotyping studies have been undertaken for the wild equids, and some variation has been noted in their karyotypes. We do not know whether the individuals studied had clinically abnormal karyotypes or whether this variation represents hybridization between chromosomally heterogeneous populations that were brought together in recent history.

Endangered species

The conservation status of the different species of *Equus* is identified on far right of Table 18.1 according to the IUCN. Those listed as critically endangered (Somali wild ass), endangered (Przewalski's horse, kulan, onager, and Grevy's zebra), and vulnerable (mountain zebra) are those considered at risk of extinction. Those identified as of least concern (kiang and common or plains zebra) are considered as stable populations for the present.

Table 18.1. Chromosome numbers found among those extant species of the Equidae that have been karyotyped. In several species, variation in chromosome number has been described and these numbers are shown. Usually, these variants appear to be simple fusions or fissions of two chromosomes. Data are compiled from information in Ryder *et al.* (1978), Benirschke and Ryder (1985), Bowling and Millon (1988), Ryder and Chemnick (1990), and Houck *et al.* (1998).

Species	Common names	Chromosome no.(2*n*)	IUCN Status
Horses			
Equus ferus przewalskii	Przewalski's wild horse, Mongolian wild horse (takhi)	66	Endangered
E. f. caballus (or *E. caballus*)	Domestic horse	64	Not applicable
Asses			
E. africanus somaliensis	Somali wild ass	62–64	Critically endangered
E. a. asinus	Domestic ass, donkey, burro	62	Not applicable
Asiatic Wild Asses			
E. hemionus onager	Persian wild ass (onager)	55, 56	Endangered
E. h. kulan	Transcaspian wild ass (kulan)	54, 55	Endangered
E. kiang	Tibetan wild ass (kiang)	51, 52	Least concern
Zebras			
E. grevyi	Grevy's zebra	46	Endangered
E. quagga burchellii	Burchell's zebra (common or plains zebra)	44	Least concern
E. zebra hartmannae	Hartmann's mountain zebra	32	Vulnerable

Genomic differences among the species of Equidae

The relationships among the species of Equidae continue to be clarified as we obtain more DNA sequence information. At the time of writing, whole genome sequences have been published for two horses (Wade *et al.*, 2009; Doan *et al.*, 2012), and we anticipate the publication of whole genome sequences for other species of Equidae as the costs of DNA sequencing decrease. Leading up to whole genome sequencing, comparative genome mapping has been conducted using a technique called "cross-species chromosome painting" or "zoo-FISH". This technique entails isolation of chromosomes or chromosome segments (probes) from one species, labeling them with fluorescent dyes, followed by hybridizing the probes to chromosomes of a second species. Regions bound by the probes show the chromosomal regions of homology between the two species. Chromosome painting has been very useful for understanding the complex chromosomal rearrangements that have occurred among the Equidae.

Horses

This group comprises two species, commonly known as Przewalski's horse and the domestic horse. The domestic horse is well known and is the primary subject of this book. The ancestor of the horse, sometimes called a tarpan (*E. ferus ferus* and *E. f. sylvestris*), has become extinct in the wild but the natural distribution was throughout modern-day Europe, Asia and the Middle East (Groves and Ryder, 2000). Przewalski's horse is a closely related species that became extinct in the wild during the 1900s, and was then repopulated to the Hustai National Park of Mongolia in 1992 using captive bred Przewalski's horses (Boyd and King, 2011). Before its initial extinction in the wild, the natural distribution of Przewalski's horses appears to have been from eastern Germany through to the northern regions of Asia, especially Mongolia. The extant Przewalski's horse population is descended from only 12 horses brought into zoo populations in the early 1900s. Today, the number of Przewalski's horses exceeds 1800, including more than 300 living in the wild.

The relationship between Przewalski's horses and domestic horses continues to be a topic of research and discussion. Whether or not they are fully separate species or subspecies of *Equus ferus*, genetic differences have been clearly defined between them (Lau *et al.*, 2009). Differences in overall genome organization are minimal, and apparently limited to a simple chromosome rearrangement in an ancestral species such that ECA5 (i.e. domestic horse chromosome 5) is homologous to the fusion of EPR23 and EPR24 (Przewalski's horse chromosomes 23 and 24) (Myka *et al.*, 2003). As the genome organization is similar for all other aspects of *E. f. caballus* and *E. f. przewalskii*, hybrid females are fertile.

Genome sequencing data suggests that prior to the capture of Przewalski's horses in the wild, some crossing occurred with domestic horses, which led to the sharing of DNA sequences for some regions. At the same time, the distribution of unique DNA sequences suggests that gene flow occurred only in the direction from the domestic horse to Przewalski's horse (Wade *et al.*, 2009). Moreover, the mitochondrial genome and the Y chromosome of Przewalski's horses and domestic horses are distinctly different (Oakenfull and Ryder, 1998; Oakenfull *et al.*, 2000; Wallner *et al.*, 2003; Lindgren *et al.*, 2004; Lau *et al.*, 2009).

Asses

Asses evolved in northern Africa. Following domestication, the donkey is found throughout the world because of its usefulness in agriculture. The Somali wild ass continues to exist in the wild in regions of Ethiopia and Eritrea. At present, the number of Somali wild asses may be less than 600 and the species is considered endangered (Moehlman *et al.*, 2008c).

The ass karyotype differs numerically from that of the horse by a single chromosome pair, but the morphology and banding patterns of the individual chromosomes are quite different from those of the horse too. Chromosome painting studies have demonstrated large numbers of rearrangements in genome organization when comparing asses with horses (Raudsepp and Chowdhary, 2001). The karyotypes of the Somali wild ass and the domestic ass cannot be distinguished. A simple chromosome polymorphism has been described several times that involves the same large metacentric chromosome (Benirschke and Ryder, 1985; Bowling and Millon, 1988). Studies of mitochondrial DNA from the extant asses and museum specimens of the extinct Nubian wild ass (*E. africanus africanus*) indicated that the domestic donkey appears to have descended from the Nubian wild ass and another unknown, ancestral species, but to be distinct from the Somali wild ass (Kimura *et al.*, 2011).

Asiatic Wild Asses

The taxonomy of the Asiatic wild asses has a considerable degree of uncertainty. They have been difficult to study because of their distribution in remote locations throughout Asia, and their scarcity in zoo collections and in the wild. While popularly referred to as kiangs, onagers, and kulans, the existence of multiple species and subspecies of Asiatic wild asses is a matter of continuing research and discussion (Groves and Ryder, 2000). The kiang has sometimes been described as being composed of three subspecies, *E. kiang kiang*, *E. k. holdereri*, and *E. k. polyodon*. Table 18.1 shows the results from karyotyping the kulan (*E. h. kulan*), the onager (*E. h. onager*), and the kiang. The kulan and onager (i.e. hemione) karyotypes are similar to each other, but differ in having extensive rearrangements when compared with African wild asses. Kiangs have from two to four fewer chromosomes than the hemiones and are genetically distinct based on studies of mitochondrial DNA (Oakenfull and Ryder, 1998; Oakenfull *et al.*, 2000). Reports of population polymorphisms for the kulan, onager, and kiang involve Robertsonian polymorphisms, probably of the same homologous elements (Ryder and Chemnick, 1990). Mitochondrial DNA sequence comparisons of *E. h. kulan* and *E. h. onager* showed minimal differences and led the authors to raise questions about designations of these animals as separate subspecies (Oakenfull and Ryder, 1998; Oakenfull *et al.*, 2000). For more information about the status of Asiatic wild asses, see Shah *et al.* (2008) and Moehlman *et al.* (2008b).

Zebras

The best-known feature of the African zebras is probably the presence of extensive, distinctive striping patterns. Despite this common characteristic, the zebra group is

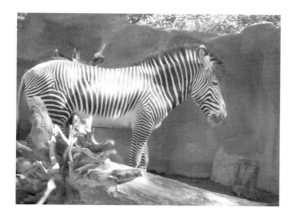

Fig. 18.3. Grevy's zebra.

genetically quite diverse. As can be seen from Table 18.1, they are typically regarded as belonging to three species groups (*E. grevyi*, *E. quagga* and *E. zebra*), and have chromosome numbers ranging from 32 to 46.

Grevy's zebra (*E. grevyi*; see Fig. 18.3) is characterized as a single species. The species is not very numerous and is classified as endangered.

Several subspecies have been described for *E. quagga*. *E. q. burchellii* has the common name of Burchell's zebra, or common or plains zebra. Other subspecies of *E. quagga* have been recognized as *E. q. boehmi* (Grant's zebra), *E. q. zambiensis*, *E. q. borensis* (maneless zebra), *E. q. chapmani* (Chapman's zebra), *E. q. crawshayi* (Crawshay's zebra), and *E. q. selousi* (Selousi's zebra). This group is denoted as of "least concern" meaning that the populations appear to be stable.

E. zebra is considered to be vulnerable and occurs in two populations: the Hartman's mountain zebra (*E. z. hartmannae*) and the Cape Mountain zebra (*E. z. zebra*).

Zebra species are also distinctive by their ranges with limited overlap, especially in modern time. Chromosome painting has been used to identify the differences in genome organization among the different species (Trifonov *et al.*, 2008). For more information, see Hack and Lorensen (2008), Moehlman *et al.* (2008a), and Novellie (2008).

Species Hybrids

Despite extensive chromosomal differences, the various equine species generally can be successfully crossed to produce viable progeny. In the late 1800s, a series of experiments was conducted to construct hybrids with zebras and horses, and were described in a book called *The Penycuik Experiments* (Ewart, 1899; now available as a digitized book). Such hybrids show that, despite extensive chromosomal and genomic changes, the overall genomic content between members within the genus *Equus* is not markedly different and viable offspring can be produced. However, the hybrids are usually sterile. During meiosis in hybrids, the chromosomes of the two parent species pair, interchange DNA, then have difficulties creating sperm or eggs with the correct amount of DNA and number of genes because of the different arrangements of the genes. For this reason, only hybrids between very closely related species, such as Przewalski's horse and the domestic horse, or among the hemiones, can produce fertile offspring.

Rare fertility in mules and hinnies

Historically, the species cross between the domestic horse and donkey has been agriculturally highly important. The offspring of a female horse and a male donkey is called a mule; the reciprocal cross between a female donkey and a male horse produces a hybrid called a hinny. Both hybrids have 63 chromosomes; 32 from the horse parent and 31 from the donkey parent. The ovaries of most female horse/donkey hybrids are usually non-functional (atrophic) and males do not produce sperm (they are azoospermic). The occurrence of fertile mules is very rare because of the failure to produce viable gametes. Some rare exceptions have been documented. Ryder *et al.* (1985) used karyotyping and blood typing to confirm the parentage of a jack (male) mule foal by a Welsh pony stallion out of a molly (female) mule. Karyotyping studies of fertile female mules and hinnies in China have also been reported (Rong *et al.*, 1988).

Feral Species

Wild species of equids have been extinct in North America for thousands of years (except for zoo collections), but feral horses and donkeys are wild and free ranging in several locations around the world. The feral animals are descended from domestic horses and asses.

References

Benirschke, K. and Ryder, O.A. (1985) Genetic aspects of equids with particular reference to their hybrids. *Equine Veterinary Journal* (Supplement 3), 1–10.

Bowling, A.T. and Millon, L. (1988) Centric fission in the karyotype of a mother–daughter pair of donkeys *(Equus asinus)*. *Cytogenetics and Cell Genetics* 47, 152–154.

Bowling, A.T., Breen, M., Chowdhary, B.P., Hirota, K., Lear, T., Millon, L.V., Ponce de Leon, F.A., Raudsepp, T. and Stranzinger, G. (1997) International system for cytogenetic nomenclature of the domestic horse: Report of the Third International Committee for the Standardization of the domestic horse karyotype, Davis, CA, USA, 1996. *Chromosome Research* 5, 433–443.

Boyd, L. and King, S.R.B. (2011) *Equus ferus*. In: IUCN (2012) IUCN Red List of Threatened Species. Version 2012.2. Available at: www.iucnredlist.org (accessed 22 January 2013).

Di Meo, G.P., Perucatti, A., Peretti, V., Incarnato, D., Ciotola, F., Liotta, L., Raudsepp, T., Di Berardino, D., Chowdhary, B. and Iannuzzi, L. (2009) The 450-band resolution G- and R-banded standard karyotype of the donkey (*Equus asinus*, 2*n* = 62). *Cytogenetic and Genome Research* 125, 266–271.

Doan, R., Cohen, N.D., Sawyer, J., Ghaffari, N., Johnson, C.D. and Dindot, S.V. (2012) Whole-genome sequencing and genetic variant analysis of a Quarter Horse mare. *BMC Genomics* 13:78, doi:10.1186/1471-2164-13-78.

Ewart, J.C. (1899) *The Penycuik Experiments*. Adam and Charles Black, London. Digitized version available at: http://archive.org/details/penycuikexperim00ewargoog (accessed 22 January 2013).

Groves, C.P. and Ryder, O.A. (2000) Systematics and phylogeny of the horse. In: Bowling, A.T. and Ruvinsky, A. (eds) *The Genetics of the Horse*. CAB International, Wallingford, UK, pp. 1–24.

Hack, M.A and Lorenzen, E. (2008) *Equus quagga*. In: IUCN (2012) IUCN Red List of Threatened Species. Version 2012.2. Available at: www.iucnredlist.org (accessed 22 January 2013).

Houck, M.L., Kumamoto, A.T., Cabrera, R.M. and Benirschke, K. (1998) Chromosomal rearrangements in a Somali wild ass pedigree, *Equus africanus somaliensis* (Perissodactyla, Equidae). *Cytogenetics and Cell Genetics* 80, 117–122.

Kimura, B. *et al.* (2011) Ancient DNA from Nubian and Somali wild ass provides insights into donkey ancestry and domestication. *Proceedings of the Royal Society B* 278(1702), 50–57.

Lau, A.N., Peng, L., Goto, H., Chemnick, L., Ryder, O.A. and Makova, K.D. (2009) Horse domestication and conservation genetics of Przewalski's horse inferred from sex chromosomal and autosomal sequences. *Molecular Biology and Evolution* 26, 199–208.

Lindgren, G., Backström, N., Swinburne, J., Hellborg, L., Einarsson, A., Sandberg, K., Cothran, G., Vilà, C., Binns, M. and Ellegren, H. (2004) Limited number of patrilines in horse domestication. *Nature Genetics* 36, 335–336.

Moehlman, P.D., Rubenstein, D.I. and Kebede, F. (2008a) *Equus grevyi*. In: IUCN (2012) IUCN Red List of Threatened Species. Version 2012.2. Available at: www.iucnredlist.org (accessed 22 January 2013).

Moehlman, P.D., Shah, N. and Feh, C. (2008b) *Equus hemionus*. In: IUCN (2012) IUCN Red List of Threatened Species. Version 2012.2. Available at: www.iucnredlist.org (accessed 22 January 2013).

Moehlman, P.D., Yohannes, H., Teclai, R. and Kebede, F. (2008c) *Equus africanus*. In: IUCN (2012) IUCN Red List of Threatened Species. Version 2012.2. Available at: www.iucnredlist.org (accessed 22 January 2013).

Myka, J.L., Lear, T.L., Houck, M.L., Ryder, O.A. and Bailey, E. (2003) FISH analysis comparing genome organization in the domestic horse (*Equus caballus*) to that of the Mongolian wild horse (*E. przewalskii*). *Cytogenetic and Genome Research* 102, 222–225.

Novellie, P. (2008) *Equus zebra*. In: IUCN (2012) IUCN Red List of Threatened Species. Version 2012.2. Available at www.iucnredlist.org (accessed 22 January 2013).

Oakenfull, E.A. and Ryder, O.A. (1998) Mitochondrial control region and 12S rRNA variation in Przewalski's horse (*Equus przewalskii*). *Animal Genetics* 29, 456–459.

Oakenfull, E.A., Lim, H.N. and Ryder, O.A. (2000) A survey of equid mitochondrial DNA: implications for the evolution, genetic diversity and conservation of *Equus*. *Conservation Genetics* 1, 341–355.

Raudsepp, T. and Chowdhary, B.P. (2001) Correspondence of human chromosomes 9, 12, 15, 16, 19 and 20 with donkey chromosomes refines homology between horse and donkey karyotypes. *Chromosome Research* 9, 623–629.

Raudsepp, T., Christensen, K. and Chowdhary, B.P. (2000) Cytogenetics of donkey chromosomes: nomenclature proposal based on GTG-banded chromosomes and depiction of NORs and telomeric sites. *Chromosome Research* 8, 659–670.

Rong, R., Chandley, A.C., Song, J., McBeath, S., Tan, P.P., Bai, Q. and Speed, R.M. (1988) A fertile mule and hinny in China. *Cytogenetics and Cell Genetics* 47, 134–139.

Ryder, O.A. and Chemnick, L.G. (1990) Chromosomal and molecular evolution in Asiatic wild asses. *Genetica* 83, 67–72.

Ryder, O.A., Epel, N.C. and Benirschke, K. (1978) Chromosome banding studies of the Equidae. *Cytogenetics and Cell Genetics* 20, 323–350.

Ryder, O.A., Chemnick, L.G., Bowling, A.T. and Benirschke, K. (1985) Male mule foal qualifies as the offspring of a female mule and jack donkey. *Journal of Heredity* 76, 379–381.

Shah, N., St Louis, A., Huibin, Z., Bleisch, W., Van Gruissen, J. and Qureshi, Q. (2008) *Equus kiang*. In: IUCN (2012) IUCN Red List of Threatened Species. Version 2012.2. Available at: www.iucnredlist.org (accessed 22 January 2013).

Trifonov, V.A. *et al.* (2008) Multidirectional cross-species painting illuminates the history of karyotypic evolution in Perissodactyla. *Chromosome Research* 16, 89–107.

Wade, C.M. *et al.* (2009) Genome sequence, comparative analysis, and population genetics of the domestic horse. *Science* 326, 865–867.

Wallner, B., Brem, G., Müller, M. and Achmann, R. (2003) Fixed nucleotide differences on the Y chromosome indicate clear divergence between *Equus przewalskii* and *Equus caballus*. *Animal Genetics* 34, 453–456.

19 Frequently Asked Questions

As an alternative format for presenting information, here are answers (A) for specific situations that are representative of frequently asked questions (Q) about horse genetics. You will have no difficulty sensing our frustration that good questions often have inadequate answers because basic genetic research data for the horse are lacking.

Color, Hair Characteristics, and Gait

Blue eyes?

Q: *I have a Welsh Pony mare that just had her third foal, all by the same stallion. Much to my surprise, one of the filly's eyes is partially blue. Neither the sire nor the dam has a blue or partial blue eye. None of the other 17 foals by this stallion has had this trait nor have the mare's other two foals. How is this trait inherited?*

A: Unfortunately, the scientific literature does not provide a definitive scheme for the inheritance of blue or partial blue eyes (heterochromia irides) in the horse. Blue eyes are a frequent feature in breeds with major spotting genes (tobiano, overo, appaloosa). They are also expected in the extreme color dilution phenotypes (cremello and perlino) where their sun sensitivity may be a significantly undesirable characteristic. Blue-eyed foals are not anticipated in breedings between non-spotted, non-dilute parents, but certainly occur in many breeds, although rarely. Blue or partial blue eyes in non-dilute colored horses do not seem to be sun sensitive or otherwise defective.

The inheritance of this characteristic does not seem to follow a simple Mendelian pattern. In most cases, neither parent of a blue-eyed foal has blue eyes, so it is not a simple dominant trait. Breeding data from blue-eyed stallions bred to brown-eyed and blue-eyed mares might be quite useful to help sort out the inheritance. These data may be difficult to obtain because the common notion is that a solid-color horse with blue eyes is undesirable and seldom would mare owners be enticed to breed to such a stallion even if he was otherwise outstanding. The inheritance of blue eyes is but one of the unanswered genetic dilemmas in breeding horses. Perhaps a breeder has some data that could be shared or would be willing to underwrite a project to investigate blue eye inheritance.

Tricolored Pinto?

Q: *My neighbor has a stallion that she advertises as a tricolored Pinto. This horse looks like a bay tobiano to me. She claims his color is very special. I can't find any discussion of this color in horse genetics books. Can you tell me more about this color?*

A: The advertisements that I have seen for "tricolored" tobianos look like either bay or buckskin tobianos. I am not aware of any special genetic situation that would give rise to these color combinations. Perhaps the point the owners are trying to make is that everyone else is keen to have a black tobiano and their horse provides an alternative.

Coat color genes?

Q: *What kind samples do I need to send to get a readout of the coat color genes of my buckskin Peruvian Paso mare?*

A: Blood samples or hair roots are the most common sources of DNA for testing for coat color genes. From your description, it seems most likely that your mare will be: *ww, gg, E–, A–, CRcr, dndn, zz, chch, toto, oo, lplp, rnrn, sb1sb1*. You can pay the laboratory to verify each of those observations. However, tests just for the *Extension* locus (*E* or *MC1R*) and for the *Agouti* locus (*A* or *ASIP*) could tell you whether or not your horse is homozygous for the *E* and *A* alleles of those loci.

Roan lethal?

Q: *I have a bay roan Quarter Horse stallion that is a many times champion cutting horse. Some people have told me I should not stand him at stud because roan is a lethal gene. He is a wonderful horse. I would like to have lots more like him and I will breed as many mares of my own as I can afford to keep. What is all this talk of roan as a lethal gene – my stallion is clearly alive.*

A: Stud book research for Belgian horses suggested that the allele for roan color is a homozygous lethal. A horse with only one copy of the allele – such as your stallion – will be healthy and obviously has no problems from having the gene. The issue only arises when using roan horses as breeding stock. Horses with two copies of the roan gene, such as could occur from breeding a roan mare to a roan stallion, allegedly die as embryos. Unfortunately, we have no direct data from breeding trials to verify this embryo lethality process. It would also be very difficult to obtain such data because of the long gestation of horses and the costs of conducting such studies. Nevertheless, many breeders and some registries have adopted practices to discourage mating roan stallions to roan mares to avoid the lowered pregnancy rate that would occur as a result of a homozygous lethal roan gene.

Anecdotal reports suggest that some roan stallions are homozygous for the gene, demonstrating that in some cases it is not lethal. The basis for the observation is that all offspring of those stallions are roan. The reports have not been verified in scientific publications, but the anecdotal reports are plausible. There could be multiple genes or mutations that cause roan color patterns, with some being homozygous lethal genes and others being compatible with homozygous viability. For example, we have discovered multiple mutations that cause the dominant white trait (Chapter 6), some of which are likely to be homozygous lethals, while others could be viable as homozygotes. We do not yet know the mutation(s) responsible for roan, but it is possible that there are multiple ways to produce a roan horse, similar to the situation for dominant white.

Lethal white in mules?

Q: *I have long been an admirer of mules. I have an overo Pinto mare that I would like to breed to my neighbor's spotted jack. Do we need to be concerned about the possibility of producing a lethal white mule?*

A: What an interesting question! Unfortunately, we have no good answer. The spotting pattern in asses, apparently inherited as a dominant trait, may be homologous to one of the spotting patterns in horses, but we are not aware of any data that provide specific details. The specific mutation that causes overo lethal white foal syndrome in horses does not occur in asses. However, a different mutation in the same gene could have a similar effect.

"True" black?

Q: *I have a black Arabian stallion with a lot of roaning on his flanks and on the top of his tail. The owner of another black stallion says my stallion is not a true black and it is improper or even unethical of me to advertise him as black. If I send you a photograph will you write a letter stating that he is a true black so that I can advertise him as such?*

A: I don't know a genetic definition for "true" black. The typical genetic situation for black is the result of the dominant gene from *Extension* and homozygosity for the recessive gene of *Agouti* (*E–aa*). The roaning trait shown by your stallion is best likened to a marking independent of the genetic basis for black. Does your nemesis also reason that a true black would have no white markings whatsoever? The problem you describe is one of the unfortunately all too common examples of breeders invoking pseudoscience to justify their personal preferences. Stand up for logic and reason, show your stallion as a performance star and advertise him as a desirable horse regardless of his color.

Curly coat?

Q: *I am the proud owner of a mustang. This special mare has a very curly hair coat. Her mane is like corkscrews. Is this an inherited trait? If yes, to what should I breed her to get a curly foal?*

A: Occasional horses with curly coats are seen in various breeds in the USA, such as the Percheron (Blakeslee *et al.*, 1943), Quarter Horse, and Missouri Fox Trotter, and they are also seen among feral horses. Stud book records of the American Bashkir Curly Registry suggest that both dominantly and recessively inherited types of curly coat may be found (Sponenberg, 2009). In my experience, the dominantly inherited type of curliness is the one found in feral horses. You can probably expect your mare to be heterozygous for the curly trait and that 50% of her foals will have a curly coat regardless of the coat type of the stallion you use.

Inheritance of ambling gait in Arabians?

Q: *My Arabian gelding is 20 years old this year. He has been a wonderful trail companion for 15 years and introduced me to the pleasures of what I call an ambling gait. He also can do the basic walk, trot, and canter repertoire, but we both prefer his four-beat amble for our pleasure rides. Am I going to be able to find another gaited Arabian to replace him or do I have to switch to a breed that has been traditionally selected for this trait?*

A: Gaited Arab horses are reported from time to time, but are certainly not common. One of the current top endurance horses is an Arabian with an amble or running walk, but we know of no one who is specifically breeding Arabian horses for this trait. We are not aware of controlled breeding trials that would define the trait inheritance pattern in Arabians. If you put a "horse wanted" ad in a national Arabian publication you will probably find several gaited horses for sale, but you are unlikely to have a large number to choose from. If you do not want to travel very far to try out a horse, you might have to switch to another breed so that you have several local examples and a wider choice of color, age, sex, and gait.

Medical Problems and Possible Genetic Disorders

Screening for defective genes?

Q: *What kind of blood samples do I need to send to identify the defective genes of a yearling Quarter Horse gelding I am thinking of buying? I am particularly concerned about defects of the feet and legs. My first mare went lame from navicular disease and I don't want a repeat of the problems I had with her.*

A: At this time, only a few genes controlling conformational traits have been identified, and these are only for fairly simple traits such as height. Numerous examples can be found of eminently successful performance horses with less than perfect conformation, but you are certainly justified to identify areas of special importance for your program. You may especially want to avoid horses that have been retired to brood stock status because of a problem with navicular disease (though they need not have offspring with this problem). Heritability estimates for navicular disease range from low to moderate values, indicating that there are at least genetic components to the disease (Diesterbeck and Distl, 2007). Conformation that predisposes to unsoundness may be difficult to spot in a young horse, so be sure to try to see the parents and ask questions about how they held up to performance trials. Good luck!

Parrot mouth

Q: *Six months ago I bought a very expensive yearling Paint colt as a stallion prospect with the guarantee that I could return him if he was genetically defective. He is starting to develop a parrot mouth and I want to send him back, but the seller says I must prove this is a genetic problem. Can you send me a signed statement that this is a genetic problem so I can get my money back?*

A: Although defective genes may affect patterns of abnormal bone growth, the inheritance of parrot mouth (brachygnathism) has not been defined. Gaughan and DeBowes (1993) report a brachygnathic sire with one affected foal out of 41, so inheritance is clearly not due to a simple dominant gene. Males are more often affected than females, another fact pointing inheritance away from a conclusion of a simple Mendelian gene. Probably parrot mouth is a polygenic trait that can be influenced by environmental components (nutrition) as well as by genes.

No laboratory tests are available to define the relative importance of each component in particular cases. In your situation, the genetic component could probably only be proven by breeding the colt to normal and affected mares to see whether and how frequently he transmitted the trait. I agree that this suggestion is not a practical solution to your problem, but at some point these studies need to be done and the results published so that sellers and buyers can be the responsible horse breeders that they want to be. Your situation emphasizes the importance of listing specific conditions in the contract that would allow you to return the colt for a refund of purchase price. Buyer protection laws in your state may help you even if you did not specify conditions in the contract. However, in most animal transactions, probably the assumption is "buyer beware". The buyer who agrees to assume unnamed risks (no guaranteed refund) may be successful in negotiating a lower price for a young, but unproven breeding prospect.

Cryptorchidism?

Q: *I am a small breeder with only two Tennessee Walking horse mares and no stallion. Every year I breed them to world champions. Last year both mares had colts by the same stallion. They are nice colts, but one is a cryptorchid as a yearling. My veterinarian cannot palpate his second testicle. I want you to help me sue the stallion owner to reimburse me for my stud fees and all my expenses in raising these foals, and to prevent him from defrauding other mare owners. He says that my colt is the only cryptorchid his stallion has sired from nearly 100 foals. My mares have each had one other colt by another stallion, but neither was a cryptorchid.*

A: Cryptorchidism is the failure of one or both testicles to descend into the scrotum. If the retained testicle is abdominal, then it is unlikely to descend, but a testicle in the inguinal canal of a young colt may later descend. Cryptorchidism is another one of those assumed genetic traits with insufficient evidence to support the popular assumption. The problem seems to occur in all breeds. It is probably an elusive polygenic trait with a threshold effect and the extra complication that trait expression is limited to males. Possibly some cases have an environmental cause (such as poor nutrition or trauma at birth or later). If this is a genetic trait, most likely your mare as well as the stallion contributed problem genes to the colt. The standard breeding contract you signed only guaranteed a foal that could stand to nurse. Perhaps you should have discussed a different set of guarantees with the stallion owner before breeding your mares.

Inheritance of HYPP?

Q: *I have a 7 year old Appaloosa mare that has tested positive for HYPP, but she has no symptoms of the disease that I have ever seen. Can she still transmit the gene if I breed her to a stallion that is negative for the HYPP gene?*

A: *HYPP* gene positive horses (*N/H*) that do not appear to have muscle paralysis episodes can transmit the defective gene. Minimally affected heterozygous *HYPP* horses may have less of the abnormal gene product than more severely affected heterozygotes (Zhou *et al.*, 1994), but we have no evidence for variability in trait transmission between minimally and severely affected heterozygotes. Diet and exercise-managed *HYPP* gene positive horses can appear to be asymptomatic but will transmit the gene to 50% of their foals regardless of the other parent.

Wobbler colt?

Q: *I have a yearling gelding by an imported Dutch Warmblood stallion out of a 16 year old Thoroughbred mare. I have used this mare very successfully in sport horse competition. Her yearling son is big, correct, handsome, and just what I was looking for to replace his mother as my competition horse. He is turned out in pasture with other yearlings and for the last month he hasn't been moving right. He is clumsy and uncoordinated. My veterinarian says he is ataxic due to a spinal cord injury of unknown origin. From what I have read, the "wobbler" problem could be caused by cervical vertebral fracture (trauma) or by vertebral malformation (possibly genetic). The stallion has lots of foals and the owner knows of no other wobblers. She has offered to rebreed my mare for free. Assuming the problem is genetic, what are my chances of getting another wobbler?*

A: As you are aware, injury has not been ruled out as the source for your colt's problem and if a fracture can be demonstrated the genetic question is a moot point for you. However, the genetic issue occurs frequently. The literature on the genetics of wobbler syndrome is contradictory in several points. It is agreed by all studies that the problem is not inherited as a simple dominant and that wobbler × wobbler matings do not produce all wobbler offspring, thus ruling out a recessive hypothesis. Males are much more often affected than females, but an affected male bred to mares who had previously produced affected offspring did not produce wobbler foals, so the problem is not due to an X-linked gene. The genetic analysis by Falco *et al.* (1976) failed to find evidence to support a genetic hypothesis for wobbler syndrome, at least for Thoroughbreds in Britain, and suggested that environmental factors should be closely examined as possible causative influences for the disease.

Prenatal testing as a tool for genetic selection in horses?

Q: *I would like to get a tobiano foal from my tobiano Paint mare. From the standpoint of conformation, I would like to breed her to my palomino Quarter Horse stallion, but I realize my chances of getting a tobiano foal are only 50%. Once the mare is pregnant, could I do any tests of her blood or maybe do amniocentesis to tell me if the foal is solid so that I could abort the pregnancy and try again for a tobiano?*

A: Prenatal testing is increasingly used in human medicine for pregnancies at risk for a deleterious genetic disease. Potentially the same kinds of procedures could be applied to horses, but practical considerations may make them unrealistic. Termination of a pregnancy in horses must occur very early in gestation so that the mare will return to cycling within a few weeks. If the embryo develops beyond about 40 days, endometrial cup formation may prevent the mare from returning to estrus for several months, so you may not get a foal for that season. Another limitation would be finding a veterinarian skilled at amniocentesis in horses, but an approach to an equine reproduction specialist would be a good place to start your inquiries.

As a DNA test for tobiano is available, embryo transplantation is another route that you might consider for your project. Several clinics nationwide provide such services for horses, although I am not aware that they are currently using genetic screening to select embryos. Using this route, you would recover an embryo from the mare soon after fertilization and test a few cells with the appropriate DNA technology. If the embryo was not of the desired genetic type, you could try again with another embryo from the mare's subsequent cycle. An acceptable embryo could be reintroduced into the donor or into any appropriate recipient mare to complete the pregnancy to term.

Carrier testing with random matings?

Q: *I am very interested in breeding my American Saddlebred mare to a young stallion that has the qualities of bone and scope she needs. This horse only has seven foals on the ground. My mare has exceptional movement and attitude, but is possibly the carrier of an autosomal recessive lethal gene. I do not want to do this breeding if the stallion carries the same gene. How many normal foals from random matings are needed to prove that a stallion is not a carrier of this defective gene?*

A: Random mating is not a very effective test of carrier status, but is often the only information available. The answer depends on the gene frequency of the trait of concern. If 20% of the population carry a gene for an autosomal recessive undesirable trait, then about 60 unaffected foals from random matings are needed to provide statistical assurance at the 95% level that the stallion is not a carrier. If the trait is rare, say a carrier frequency of 2%, then 600 unaffected foals from random matings would be needed for 95% statistical assurance of non-carrier status of the sire.

Preventing NI problems?

Q: *I own a pregnant Thoroughbred mare that I purchased 2 years ago. Her previous owners told me she had lost a foal to neonatal isoerythrolysis (NI). How can I have her tested to see if this foal is at risk? Can you also help me find a stallion that I can breed her to so I won't have to worry about NI at all?*

A: A serum sample from the pregnant mare taken about 3 weeks before she is due to foal can be screened to see if a blood group incompatibility is detected that could lead to destruction of the foal's red blood cells (RBCs) and its death. If the test results are positive for anti-blood group activity, you should be prepared to attend the birth of the foal, making certain the foal does not suckle its dam and providing it with an alternative colostrum source. The foal can be put back to its dam's milk after 36–48 h.

To prevent the problem in future foals, you can try to locate a stallion negative for the problem blood group factor. For example, if the mare has anti-Aa antibodies, you could anticipate no NI problems in subsequent foals if the mare is bred to a stallion lacking the Aa factor. However, the Aa factor is very common, and it may be difficult to find a stallion that lacks it and would suit in other ways. If the problem is Qa (or any other specificity), it will probably not be as difficult to find a blood-group compatible stallion. It may not be possible to find a stallion that is also suitable in pedigree, location, stud fee, and conformation. In that case, you will need to manage the newborn foal as outlined above.

Infertility in a filly born co-twin to a colt?

Q: *I have a yearling Quarter Horse filly that was twin to a colt that died at birth. My father tells me that in cattle, heifers born co-twin to bull calves are nearly always infertile. Is this also a possibility for horses?*

A: This cattle condition is called "freemartinism". The biological mechanism that produces the freemartin is not known, but it is related to the masculinizing effect of shared blood circulation between twins of unlike sex that renders the heifer sterile. Evidence of shared circulation in horse twins has been reported from studies of fetal membranes after birth and confirmed by blood group chimerism and mixed XX/XY karyotypes from blood cultures of twin-born horses of unlike sex, but no cases of a masculinizing effect on the filly have been reported.

We have looked for a freemartin effect in horses using stud book data provided by the Arabian Horse Registry of America. We compared registrations for foals from twin-born mares in a female–female (FF) pair with foals from mares in a male–female (MF) pair. Among the 35 MF pairs occurring up to registration number 200,000 (foaling date up to about 1978), 24 mares had registered foals and 11 had none. Among the 19 FF twin pairs (38 mares), 30 had registered foals and eight had none. The difference between these groups is not statistically significant.

So the available evidence seems to be that the freemartin effect found in cattle is not of major concern for horse breeders. Infertility is not expected for a filly born co-twin to a colt.

Parentage Testing, Relatedness and Pedigrees

Deriving genetic markers for a dead horse?

Q: *My Morgan mare died before I had her parentage tested. To register her foal I need to verify its parentage to both the dam and the sire. I have two full sisters to that foal. Can the type of the unregistered foal be compared with theirs to satisfy the parentage verification requirements?*

A: Two offspring of an untested parent are insufficient to define the allelic pairs for the standard set of microsatellite DNA markers. To derive the genetic type of a dead horse at least 15–20 offspring are usually needed. Fewer offspring may be sufficient if their other parent or the parents of the dead horse can be tested.

If the dead mare was buried, it is possible that DNA testing from teeth or bone can be used to obtain a genetic profile for direct parentage validation. Be sure to check with your registrar to see what kinds of genetic testing evidence is acceptable. He/she may help you access other genetic records that could help your derivation project.

Preservation of breeding lines and genetic diversity?

Q: *My family has raised registered Arabian horses on our cattle ranch for about 50 years. My grandfather read extensively about the history and tradition of Arab horse breeding before selecting his horses from England and related horses from the USA. My uncle worked as an oil geologist in Saudi Arabia and brought back two mares from there for my father's breeding program. Now I am in line to direct this program. I took a degree in English history, without training in science or genetics. I do not want to change these horses. They suit our needs. Although we have never taken a horse to a show, a couple that we have sold have competed successfully both in the show ring and in performance. Most of our horses are in some degree related to each other and perhaps it is time to add new breeding stock. I have been reading Arabian horse magazines and have visited some "big-name" stables but I do not feel that the current show horse Arabian is what my grandfather had in mind when he set up our program. Am I right in thinking that I can preserve our stock as a genetically healthy group of Arabians without joining the mainstream?*

A: Modern animal science principles encourage the selection of breeding stock based on measured excellence (racing speed, show championships, milk production, egg production, and so on). For your program, such criteria may not be predictors of excellence. As your horses suit your family's needs, you are certainly justified to stay with them. Your group is relatively little inbred at the moment and you may not need to add outside stock to maintain the program for many more years. If you did want to add horses, one possibility may be to find horses related to your grandfather's early imports from England or your uncle's more recent desert imports.

We cannot know what uses will be made of horses in the future, but 20th century history has shown that narrow specialization can doom a breed. It is important to maintain diversity even in – or particularly in – the context of closed stud books. Preservation programs are providing a strong voice for conserving breeding options. You are in a prime position to contribute to and benefit from such movements. If you choose this route for your breeding program, be prepared for skepticism from mainstream breeders, but be assured that the genetic basis is no less valid in the long-term view than a program based on racetrack or arena winnings.

Genetic reconstruction of a highly regarded stallion?

Q: *I hope your genetic marker testing can help me to breed a genetic replica of a wonderful old Quarter Horse stallion that died 2 years ago. I have a daughter of this horse. I understand that she only got half of his chromosomes. Could your tests help me find a son for breeding with my mare that got the alternative chromosomes? I know I may have to repeat the mating several times and I know that my chances are not 100% to exactly match the old horse. The books say you need to use the young stallions to make genetic progress, but for my program the old-time genes are just fine and I can consistently produce just the kind of horse I need.*

A: Unfortunately, the Grand Genetic Game Plan is working against you in any scheme to *breed* a clone of the old stallion. As you know, the old stallion could only contribute half his genes to each foal. Your goal would be a double grandson to which its parents transmitted all the genes they received from the old stallion and none of the genes they received from their dams. Even if you could find a son of this old stallion that received the "other half" of his genes than your mare did, it is probably impossible for you to raise enough foals from them to meet the statistical challenge of your proposal.

Genetic planning is clearly possible at the level of selection for a few genes where the genetics is defined, such as breeding for certain coat colors. For conformation and performance traits, where the genetics is much less defined and hundreds or thousands of genes are involved, the outcomes are much less predictable. Your skill as a breeder is determined by luck as well as an intuitive understanding of the breeding consistencies of horses familiar to you. Science can help you to plan matings for simple defined traits and predict the probabilities of the various outcomes, but the larger picture is still up to your vision.

Finding an identity for a rescued horse?

Q: *I purchased a mare from the Society for the Prevention of Cruelty to Animals that had been rescued from a situation of poor care and near starvation. She is said to be a registered Morgan, but we do not have any specific details. She is bay with a star, about 10 years old. Could you look at her genetic markers and tell me who she is so I can get the papers for her?*

A: You need to work with the American Morgan Horse Association (AHMA) to see what would be possible under their rules and regulations. If the AMHA considered the project to be appropriate, the Morgan database could be searched to look for a horse with genetic markers that match those of your horse. Of course, age, sex, color, and white markings would need to match as well. Even if a complete match were found, you would need to convince them beyond a shadow of a doubt that this is not a coincidence. Such an application of tests for genetic markers goes beyond the original design of the tests, which were set up to detect horses that were incorrectly presented as products of a particular set of parents. There is a subtle but significant difference between these two applications. The tests have value for identification of horses but this particular application would set a precedent.

Cloning

Q: *Would a clone of Secretariat win the Kentucky Derby?*

A: Secretariat is one of the most recognized names among Thoroughbred racehorses. He was a phenomenal 3 year old colt that won the American Triple Crown in 1973. Many consider him to be the best Thoroughbred racehorse of all time.

Scientists can now clone horses. However, cloning can only be done using viable cells. Secretariat passed away and there are no viable cells of his to use for cloning. While this makes the question moot, we can use this example for a "thought experiment".

So, would a clone of Secretariat be another super racehorse? Secretariat was probably the perfect example of his genetic type. But chance events during development, such as the number of times a cell divides, or how far it migrates in the developing embryo, are not under strict genetic control. For example, competitive drive may be enhanced when a particular brain cell divides 200 times rather than 100 times, but the number of divisions may be a chance event during embryonic development and not strictly determined by genes. It may be that during the development of Secretariat, every progenitor cell in the brain, skeletal muscle, heart, and lungs divided and migrated just the right distance. He came to our attention because everything from genetics, development, management, and racing happened just right.

So, would ten clones of Secretariat, raised and trained the same, cross the finish line together in record time? Almost certainly not! Even if genetics, management, and racing are exactly the same for all ten, the chance events that happen during development would result in small differences, and these would be significant in winning.

References

Blakeslee, L.H., Hudson, R.S. and Hunt, H.R. (1943) Curly coat in horses. *Journal of Heredity* 34, 115–118.

Diesterbeck, U. and Distl, O. (2007) Review of genetic aspects of radiological alterations in the navicular bone of the horse. *Deutsche Tierärztliche Wochenschrift* 114, 404–411.

Falco, M.J., Whitwell, K. and Palmer, A.C. (1976) An investigation into the genetics of 'wobbler disease' in Thoroughbred horses in Britain. *Equine Veterinary Journal* 8, 165–169.

Gaughan, E.M. and De Bowes, R.M. (1993) Congenital diseases of the equine head. *Veterinary Clinics of North America: Equine Practice* 9, 93–110.

Sponenberg, D.P. (2009) *Equine Color Genetics*, 3rd edn. Wiley-Blackwell, Ames, Iowa.

Zhou, J., Spier, S.J., Beech, J. and Hoffman, E.P. (1994) Pathophysiology of sodium channelopathies: correlation of normal/ mutant mRNA ratios with clinical phenotype in dominantly inherited periodic paralysis. *Human Molecular Genetics* 3, 1599–1603.

20 Where Do We Go From Here?

If you like using a hammer, every problem looks like a nail. Geneticists are suspected of regarding all traits as hereditary. Up to a point, this is true. For example, the number of horse legs is determined by genes; however, all horses have four legs so the genetic effect is of no consequence to breeders. The real question is whether the genetic effect shows variation *and* rises to a level of significance. Is it useful? Genetics involves three basic questions:

1. How can you measure the trait?
2. Does the trait show variation?
3. Is the variation hereditary?

The foregoing chapters describe the successes that scientists have had in applying their "hammer". But scientists are also cautious. Science does not allow assumptions, but rather, rests on experimental proofs. Even so, the future of horse genetics rests with the assessments and applications made by breeders. We should ask: "How might horse breeders apply new genetic tools?"

Horse breeders have always been successful by taking advantage of technology when it arises. Pedigree records are a technology used for millennia by Arabian horse breeders and, more recently (in the 1700s!), by the British to establish the Thoroughbred horse breed. Today, veterinarians use X-rays, MRI (magnetic resonance imaging) scans, vaccines, antibiotics, and many other treatments to improve the health and welfare of horses. Horse owners have improved harnesses, saddles, sulkies, and wagons to improve riding, racing, and hauling. During the last few decades, horse owners have had access to artificial insemination, embryo transfer, and even cloning to assist reproduction. Horsemen will not be shy about adopting molecular genetics tools if they improve health, well-being, and performance.

Parentage Testing

In many respects, pedigrees are a proxy for genetics. Breeders recognize that offspring tend to be like parents. Therefore, a young, untried horse with a good pedigree is more valuable than an untried horse without a pedigree. Initially, pedigrees were based on trust and integrity among breeders, but we do know that errors occurred. Foals would switch mares in the field. Mares were sometimes inadvertently exposed to precocious colts. In some cases, devious individuals might misrepresent their stock. In short, pedigrees are powerful but imperfect. Blood typing and DNA typing provided an objective approach to verifying the veracity of each stated parentage, and parentage testing dramatically improved the integrity of the pedigree record.

The advantages of DNA testing are described in Chapter 12 in relation to medical genetics. We anticipate that future technological improvements will reduce costs, and may even provide genetic information about traits that breeders value, such as coat colors or diseases. We are just beginning to understand the genetic basis of such traits, and it will take time for us to learn how to assess valued traits using DNA tests. So pedigrees and parentage testing will provide the foundation of our registries and breeding programs for the immediate future. However, as pedigrees are merely proxies for genetics, will the endpoint be the use of genetic tests in place of pedigrees?

Health and Hereditary Diseases

This seems an obvious area of application for genetic testing. Before the development of such testing, the discovery of a hereditary disease gene in a member of a breeding line raised suspicions about the wisdom of using that line. Breeders were forced to balance potential genetic gain versus complete economic loss if the market rejected their livestock. As a consequence, breeders were justifiably cautious about revealing potential problems. Infectious diseases, accident, and bad luck are more common sources of health problems among foals than are genetic defects, but if suspicion of heritable problems arises, breeders can see the market value of their livestock plummet. Therefore, it is fortunate that today we can demand that the suspicion of a hereditary disease be verified using very specific diagnostic molecular tests.

Tests have already been developed for more than a dozen hereditary diseases and work continues to uncover more, so we will have the capacity to ensure that horses are not born with many lethal diseases or any other diseases that render them unwanted. Equally important, we will be able to verify or dismiss concerns about hereditary causes of disease through tests or simple research investigations. Yet in most cases, the use of these tests is not compulsory. It is the responsibility of the breeder to diligently apply the diagnostics to prevent unnecessary suffering of diseased foals and, sometimes, even to cull their own breeding stock in order to ensure the genetic health of the breed as a whole.

Color

Horse breeders have probably selected for variation in hair color since the beginning of domestication. When the horse genome was being investigated, coat color genes were among the first that were identified using molecular tests. This occurred because the genetics of coat color were well known for horses, which provided an excellent starting point to test the power and accuracy of the genome tools that had been developed. As described in Chapters 4–10, we can explain the basis for most coat color patterns and predict the possible colors for foals of different matings. This provides some certainty. Many of the genes responsible for coat color variation in horses were the same as those causing coat color variation in other species (*KIT*, *MITF*, *MC1R*, etc.). Yet there were some surprises. For example, the gene for gray in horses does not have this effect in other species. Furthermore, the hereditary basis of sabino, dominant white, and splashed white were each shown to have more than one genetic cause.

What remains to be discovered? Many things. We do not know what causes the intensity of pigmentation that distinguishes liver chestnuts from sorrels. While we know the genetic basis for leopard patterns, we do not know why they can appear in so many different forms. We do not know what causes the precise distribution of white for any of the white hair color patterns (tobiano, sabino, splashed white, overo, etc.). We do not know what controls the age-related changes in color patterns, especially those associated with graying. In short, as long as we are able to make distinctions among horses for color patterns, we will have targets for genetic research.

Performance

Genetic controls of performance traits are likely to be complex. If they were simple, we would have fixed them ("fixed" means that all horses would have the same genes) already by genetic selection. In some cases, there may be multiple genetic ways to achieve the same genetic potential. For example, we know that an allele of *MSTN* is associated with superior sprinting performance, although many champion sprinters do not have that allele. They must have other genes that also confer superior racing capability. Likewise, conformation is going to be a consequence of multiple genetic factors in addition to the already established nutritional factors. The complexity and interplay between genetics and environment is likely to frustrate the concept of the "perfect" genotype. Nevertheless, the informed horse owner will be able to integrate genetic potential, management, and training maximize the potential of every horse. We have a lot to learn in this area.

Genetics and Breed

Horses from the same breed look alike. This is not surprising because they are selected to look alike and share ancestors. Even a novice can distinguish most Arabian horses from most Quarter Horses. The differences are also reflected in their DNA. As horses within a breed share ancestors, they also share DNA sequences that are absent or less common among other breeds. Geneticists use this information to construct genetic trees showing the relationships among breeds. This is discussed in Chapter 17. The information can even be used to assess whether or not a horse belongs to a particular population. However, it is a statistical argument and not a statement of fact. What is the statistical power that one would accept as proof? In many respects, this use may be in validating historical records.

Will it become possible to determine the breed of a horse based on its DNA sequence? The cost of DNA sequencing is plummeting, and it seems likely that we will be able to make increasingly accurate determinations of ancestry. We need to discuss what statistical power we want to use for proof, and this question actually goes to the root of our purposes in genetic selection and breed formation. We use breeds and pedigrees as proxies for genes. We also love the history of our horses. As we become able to select genes directly, then issues of pedigree, inbreeding, and outcrossing may become secondary to direct measures of genetic constitution.

Genetics and Infectious Diseases

This book does not include a chapter on "Genetics and Infectious Diseases", although this topic is likely to become one of the most important applications of genetics within the next 20 years. We have an impending health crisis for all species because antibiotics and anthelmintic drugs are becoming less effective as pathogens develop resistance to these therapies. Genetic studies may suggest alternatives to antibiotics and anthelmintics, and even provide insights for improvement of vaccines.

Most of us take antibiotics and anthelmintic drugs for granted, though these drugs transformed healthcare less than 100 years ago. Vaccines, in contrast, have been around for several hundreds of years, initially protecting people from smallpox, and more recently from polio, influenza, tetanus, and a host of other diseases. Not too long ago, we believed that vaccines, antibiotics, and drugs would make infectious diseases a problem of the past. Unfortunately, that conclusion was premature.

We are seeing bacteria and parasites becoming resistant to antibiotic and drug treatments. These drugs were effective because they attacked a characteristic of those pathogens that was not present in mammalian cells. The drugs killed the pathogens but did not harm the host. Unfortunately, antibiotics and anthelmintics did not kill all bacteria and parasites. Rare individual bacteria and parasites had mutations that rendered them immune to the drugs, so even if the treatments killed billions of pathogens, these few individuals survived and thrived. They gave rise to the antibiotic-resistant strains of bacteria and drug-resistant parasites that plague modern generations of horses. We will need to develop new strategies to effectively prevent and treat these pathogenic diseases in the next century.

Conversely, vaccines have been very effective for some diseases but ineffective for others. Vaccination stimulates the immune system and may render it capable of fighting off viral or bacterial infections. However, some pathogens are not deterred by conventional vaccinations. The immune system is complex and protection depends upon activation of the right set of cells. These pathogens are adapted to the horse and have sometimes evolved mechanisms to evade the immune system. Consequently, we do not have effective vaccines to protect foals from strangles or foal pneumonia. Our herpesvirus vaccines only produce short-term immunity in horses. In summary, we need more information about the interaction between viruses and the horse in order to be successful.

Genetics, and especially genomics, are now being used to understand the interplay between the biology of the pathogen and the biology of the horse. If we identify horses resistant to pathogens, we can learn a useful strategy for resistance. Genetic resistance represents an experiment of nature, and will lead us to new vaccines and therapies to replace antibiotics and anthelmintics.

Summary

Horse breeders were long recognized as expert practitioners of genetics long before the insights of Gregor Mendel and Watson and Crick. This truth is reflected in the diversity of extant horse breeds as well as in the spirited competitions seen at horse shows and on racetracks. Regardless of advances in molecular genetics, the value of a horse will continue to be determined by performance and not in a test tube.

Genomic studies thus far reveal complexity that confounds any thoughts of creating designer horses. We have no capacity to deal with genetic interactions that involve 2.43 billion DNA bp, over 20,000 genes, and millions of regulatory elements. But genetic discoveries do provide us with useful insights and the ability to make simple but important decisions. A breeder of Arabian horses might like to determine that a breeding prospect is not a carrier of *SCID* and advertise that information. Someone purchasing an athletic but solid colored Appaloosa might like to test the horse for the presence of the *LP* gene. Over time, we will discover diverse ways to enhance our selection for gait, speed, endurance, and power using DNA testing.

The key will be the marketplace. New tests will appear. Breeders will choose whether or not to use them to improve their livestock. Informed buyers will choose whether or not to purchase horses by using genetic tests in association with visual assessments, radiographs, pedigree records, and performance evaluations. At present, no single method of assessment provides the complete answer needed by breeders and buyers. That answer is still found on the back of the horse.

Index